Lecture Notes on Data Engineering and Communications Technologies

Volume 60

Series Editor

Fatos Xhafa, Technical University of Catalonia, Barcelona, Spain

The aim of the book series is to present cutting edge engineering approaches to data technologies and communications. It will publish latest advances on the engineering task of building and deploying distributed, scalable and reliable data infrastructures and communication systems.

The series will have a prominent applied focus on data technologies and communications with aim to promote the bridging from fundamental research on data science and networking to data engineering and communications that lead to industry products, business knowledge and standardisation.

Indexed by SCOPUS, INSPEC.

All books published in the series are submitted for consideration in Web of Science.

More information about this series at http://www.springer.com/series/15362

K. C. Santosh · Amit Joshi
Editors

COVID-19: Prediction, Decision-Making, and its Impacts

Springer

Editors
K. C. Santosh
The University of South Dakota
Vermillion, SD, USA

Amit Joshi
Global Knowledge Research Foundation
Ahmedabad, India

ISSN 2367-4512 ISSN 2367-4520 (electronic)
Lecture Notes on Data Engineering and Communications Technologies
ISBN 978-981-15-9681-0 ISBN 978-981-15-9682-7 (eBook)
https://doi.org/10.1007/978-981-15-9682-7

This Springer imprint is published by the registered company Springer Nature Singapore Pte Ltd.
The registered company address is: 152 Beach Road, #21-01/04 Gateway East, Singapore 189721, Singapore

Preface

The book aims to outline the issues of AI and COVID-19, involving predictions, medical support decision-making, and possible impact on human life. Starting with major COVID-19 issues and challenges, it takes possible AI-based solutions for several problems, such as public health surveillance, early (epidemic) prediction, COVID-19 positive case detection, and robotics integration against COVID-19. Beside mathematical modeling, it includes the necessity of changes in innovations and possible COVID-19 impacts. The book covers a clear understanding of AI-driven tools and techniques, where pattern recognition, anomaly detection, machine learning, and data analytics are considered. It aims to include the wide range of audiences from computer science and engineering to healthcare professionals.

In total, the book is composed of 14 chapters. The first 10 chapters are related to prediction, screening, and decision-making. The remaining 4 chapters cover possible COVID-19 impacts.

In Chapter "Artificial Intelligence (AI) Joins the Fight Against COVID-19", authors discuss on how AI can be used to analyze the clinical and social patterns due to COVID-19 outbreak and help fight against COVID-19 (or related pandemics).

In Chapter "AI for Covid-19: Conduits for Public Health Surveillance", authors address the importance and/or need of AI for COVID-19 when public health into account. Authors took two case studies: Australia and Canada in their assessments.

In Chapter "A Pre-screening Approach for COVID 19 Testing based on Belief Rule-Based Expert System", authors study belief rule-based tool to detect the likelihood of COVID-19 positive cases.

In Chapter "Local Analytical System for Early Epidemic Detection", authors develop a tool that is useful for detecting early epidemic event(s), where faster analytical tools are discussed.

In Chapter "Implementing Early Detection System for Covid-19 Using Anomaly Detection", authors provide a tool that can detect early symptoms by using anomaly detection techniques. The core idea of the chapter is to provide implementation details on anomaly detector (an interactive tool) for COVID-19.

In Chapter "Covid-19 Classification Based on Gray-Level Co-occurrence Matrix and Support Vector Machine", authors used 148 chest CT images to detect possible

COVID-19 positive cases by taking 10-fold cross-validation into account. It definitely brings an idea on how CT images can be used to detect COVID-19 positive cases.

In Chapter "Rough Sets in COVID-19 to Predict Symptomatic Cases", authors study an interesting idea on rough sets theory to study inadequate knowledge (incomplete information). In their study, the primary study is to work is to minimize the number of symptoms of COVID-19 by rough set theory approach for better decision making. This symptoms-based prediction could help us while checking patients and decision-makers could be benefited while making policies and guidelines.

In Chapter "COVID-19 Detection via Wavelet Entropy and Biogeography-Based Optimization", authors experimented on chest CT images (132 patients) by taking Wavelet Entropy-based features and Biogeography-based Optimization as training algorithm.

In Chapter "Machine Learning in Fighting Pandemics: A COVID-19 Case Study", authors discuss on how machine learning can be employed for any pandemics, and they consider COVID-19, a case study.

In Chapter "Healthcare Robots to Combat COVID-19", authors review an advancement in robotic technologies and their usefulness in healthcare systems as we consider that healthcare robots are expected to assists medical experts and/or healthcare professionals (both in hospital and non-hospital settings). Further, this chapter provides an overview of various types of assistive robots employed for healthcare services especially in fighting pandemic and natural disasters

In Chapter "COVID-19: A Necessity for Changes and Innovations", authors reported the need for changes and required innovations, where traditional/conventional tools/techniques may not offer enough luxury to find solutions. In other words, data-driven AI tools/techniques are must.

In Chapter "Prediction to Service Delivery: AI in Action", authors consider the need of AI and automation with respect to COVID-19, to increase productivity. In other words, the chapter aims to throw light on how this technology is being leveraged with a special emphasis on how AI is revolutionizing Education 4.0.

In Chapter "COVID-19 Impacts Construction Industry: Now, then and Future", authors highlight the impact of novel Coronavirus on the construction industry associated with risk assessment and on how to implement the safety measures for the workers during and post pandemic.

In Chapter "COVID-19 on Air Quality Index (AQI): A Necessary Evil?", authors study the impact of COVID-19 on AQI. In their chapter unlike so many unprecedented disastrous effects happening across the world, AQI has been improved due to halt on constant air polluting activities. Authors call it "a necessary evil" as it is happening for a good reason. In their assessment, they analyze the variation in AQI by taking United States, Brazil, India, Australia, China, and Taiwan into account. This chapter brings an optimism in human lives, which we call 'silver-lining'.

South Dakota, USA — K. C. Santosh
Ahmedabad, India — Amit Joshi

Contents

Editors and Contributors

About the Editors

Dr. K. C. Santosh, Ph.D. (IEEE Senior Member) is the Chair and an Associate Professor of the and Graduate Program Director at the Department of Computer Science at the University of South Dakota (USD). Before joining USD, Dr. Santosh worked as a Research Fellow at the US National Library of Medicine (NLM), National Institutes of Health (NIH). He worked as a Postdoctoral Research Scientist at the LORIA Research Centre, Universite de Lorraine, in direct collaboration with ITESOFT, France. He also served as a Research Scientist at the INRIA Nancy Grand Est Research Centre, France, where he has received his Ph.D. diploma in Computer Science. Dr. Santosh has published more than 70 peer-reviewed research articles, 100 conference proceedings, and 11 book chapters. He has authored books, and edited 3 books, 14 journal issues, and 6 conference proceedings. He is currently Editor-In-Chief of IJSIP and an Associate Editor for several journals, such as International Journal of Machine Learning and Cybernetics and IEEE Access. He has also chaired more than 10 international conference events. His research projects have been funded by multiple agencies, including the SDCRGP, Department of Education (DOE), and the National Science Foundation (NSF). Dr. Santosh is the proud recipient of the Presidents Research Excellence Award (USD, 2019) and an award from the Department of Health & Human Services (2014).

Dr. Amit Joshi, Ph.D. is currently the Director of Global Knowledge Research Foundation, also an Entrepreneur & Researcher who has completed his master's and research in the areas of cloud computing and cryptography in medical imaging. Dr. Joshi has an experience of around 10 years in academic and industry in prestigious organizations. Dr. Joshi is an active member of ACM, IEEE, CSI, AMIE, IACSIT, Singapore, IDES, ACEEE, NPA, and many other professional societies. Currently, Dr. Joshi is the International Chair of InterYIT at International Federation of Information Processing (IFIP, Austria). He has presented and published more than 50 papers in national and international journals/conferences of IEEE and ACM. Dr. Joshi has also edited more than 40 books which are published by Springer, ACM, and other reputed publishers. Dr. Joshi has also organized more than 50 national and international conferences and programs in association with ACM, Springer, and IEEE to name a few across different including India, UK, Europe, USA, Canada, Thailand, Egypt, and many more.

Contributors

Shamim Al Mamun Institute of Information Technology, Jahangirnagar University, Savar, Dhaka, Bangladesh

Tanvi Arora Department of Computer Science and Engineering, CGC College of Engineering Landran, Mohali, India

Meenakshi S. Arya Department of CSE, SRM Institute of Science and Technology, Chennai, India

Haribhau R. Bhapkar MIT School of Engineering, Department of Mathematics, MIT ADT University's, Pune, Maharashtra, India

Debasish Biswas Department of Business Administration, Vidyasagar University, Midnapore, West Bengal, India

Ankit Chaudhary Department of Computer Science and Engineering, Bharati Vidyapeeth's College of Engineering, Delhi, India

Mohamed Chawki Visiting Professor, Aix-Marseille University, Aix-en-Provence, France

Yihao Chen School of Informatics, University of Leicester, Leicester, UK

S. Prasanna Devi Department of CSE, SRM Institute of Science and Technology, Chennai, India

Ankita Dhar Department of Computer Science, West Bengal State University, Kolkata, India

Vedika Gupta Department of Computer Science and Engineering, Bharati Vidyapeeth's College of Engineering, Delhi, India

Ji Han School of Informatics, University of Leicester, Leicester, UK;
School of Computer Science and Technology, Henan Polytechnic University, Jiaozuo, Henan, People's Republic of China

J. Hardy Lifeguard Digital Health, Vancouver, Canada

Nikita Jain Department of Computer Science and Engineering, Bharati Vidyapeeth's College of Engineering, Delhi, India

M. Shamim Kaiser Institute of Information Technology, Jahangirnagar University, Savar, Dhaka, Bangladesh

Mugunthan Karunamoorthy Executive - RPA Developer at Ernest and Young, Colombo, Sri Lanka

Yumnam Kirani CDAC, Silchar, Assam, India

N. Lilley BC Emergency Health Services, Provincial Health Services Authority, Vancouver, Canada

Parikshit N. Mahalle Department of Computer Engineering, Smt. Kashibai Navale College of Engineering, Pune, Maharashtra, India;
Department of Communication, Media and Information Technologies, Aalborg University, Copenhagen, Denmark

Mufti Mahmud Department of Computing and Technology, Nottingham Trent University, Clifton, Nottingham, UK

Soumi Majumder Department of Business Administration, Vidyasagar University, Midnapore, West Bengal, India

Himadri Mukherjee Department of Computer Science, West Bengal State University, Kolkata, India

Sk. Md. Obaidullah Department of Computer Science and Engineering, Aliah University, Kolkata, India

Kaushik Roy Department of Computer Science, West Bengal State University, Kolkata, India

K. C. Santosh Department of Computer Science, University of South Dakota, Vermillion, SD, USA

Gitanjali R. Shinde Department of Computer Engineering, Smt. Kashibai Navale College of Engineering, Pune, Maharashtra, India

Yumnam Jayanta Singh NIELIT, Guwahati, Assam, India

Yumnam Somananda Singh Assam Don Bosco University, Guwahati, Assam, India

Rituraj Soni Department of Computer Science and Engineering, Engineering College Bikaner, Bikaner, Rajasthan, India

Rishikesan Srikusan AMIESL, The Institute of Engineers Sri Lanka, Colombo, Sri Lanka

Marzia Hoque Tania Department of Engineering Science, Institute of Biomedical Engineering, University of Oxford, Headington, Oxford, UK

C. Unnithan Public Health, Torrens University, Adelaide, Australia

Xujing Yao School of Informatics, University of Leicester, Leicester, UK; Department of Medical Imaging, The Fourth People's Hospital of Huai'an, Huai'an, Jiangsu, China

Artificial Intelligence (AI) Joins the Fight Against COVID-19

Mohamed Chawki

Abstract The very first novel coronavirus case (COVID-19) was found in China in December 2019. The COVID-19 pandemic has since spread to over 215 countries and areas in the world and has significantly affected every aspect of our daily lives. At the time of writing of this chapter, the numbers of cases and deaths were still increasing significantly and showing no sign of a well-controlled situation. To illustrate, as of July 24, 2020, a cumulative total of 15,839,649 COVID-19 cases had been reported around the world. There is no doubt that artificial intelligence (AI) can be an effective tool for rapidly developing diagnostic and therapeutic modalities for new diseases and outbreaks. In this chapter, the author outlines the myriad ways in which AI can be used to analyze the clinical and social patterns of a COVID-19 outbreak and prepare society to fight against this or other pandemics in a more effective way, such as monitoring treatments and research and development of drugs and vaccines for COVID-19.

Keywords Artificial Intelligence (AI) · AI applications · COVID-19 · Coronavirus pandemic · Future of artificial intelligence

1 Introduction

The COVID-19 disease, caused by the SARS-CoV-2 virus, was identified in December 2019 in China and declared a global pandemic by the WHO on March 11 [1, 9]. The strong ability of the virus to spread among humans, its severe symptoms, its high mortality rate in high-risk populations, and the low immunity that it triggers have raised fear in all countries. Therefore, strict social distancing rules and lockdown measures were imposed, resulting in a reduction of human resources in the public health sector worldwide. This revealed the need for artificial intelligence

---

M. Chawki (✉)
Visiting Professor, Aix-Marseille University, Aix-en-Provence, France
e-mail: chawki@cybercrime-fr.org

K. C. Santosh and A. Joshi (eds.), *COVID-19: Prediction, Decision-Making, and its Impacts*, Lecture Notes on Data Engineering and Communications Technologies 60, https://doi.org/10.1007/978-981-15-9682-7_1

(AI) tools, not to replace humans, but to safely support them in their fight against COVID-19.

AI is a potentially powerful tool in the fight against the COVID-19 pandemic. AI can, for the present purposes, be defined as machine learning (ML), natural language processing (NLP), and computer vision applications to teach computers to use Big Data-based models for pattern recognition, explanation, and prediction. Several publications have dealt with potential applications of AI, particularly the ability of AI to recognize (diagnose), predict, and explain (treat) COVID-19 infections, as well as to help manage socioeconomic impacts (ibid). Since the outbreak of the pandemic, there has been a scramble to use AI and other data analytic tools for these purposes Broad [2], Hollister [7], Taulli [15]. In this chapter, the author provides a thorough review of this AI scramble, where he discusses collectively the actual and potential contributions of AI to the fight against COVID-19. The cost of the pandemic in terms of lives and economic damage will be terrible, at the time of writing, great uncertainty surrounded estimates of just how terrible and of how successful both non-pharmaceutical and pharmaceutical responses can be (ibid). As an evidence-based medical tool, AI has the potential to improve the planning, treatment, and reported outcomes of the COVID-19 patient.

2 Main Applications of AI in the COVID-19 Pandemic

AI can be used in the fight against COVID-19 in several ways: (i) smart screening for high body temperature, (ii) disease surveillance, (iii) monitoring treatment, (iv) multi-purpose platforms, (v) treatments, and cures, and (vi) development of drugs and vaccines.

2.1 Smart Screening for High Body Temperature

A mobile app with AI that assesses the risk level of users at home or anywhere else is a thin line of defense relying on the honesty of the users who answer the questions truthfully. In some busy public places, like airports, train stations, office buildings, schools, and hospitals, mass screening to try to detect visitors experiencing symptoms of COVID-19 is necessary [6]. High body temperature is one of the most common symptoms of COVID-19. Decades ago, traditional thermal scanning technology checked users one by one as they moved sequentially in a queue and stopped in front of the camera for a second or so to ensure accurate detection. Recent infrared thermal image scanner (ITIS) technology has been widely deployed at border control stations for mass screening of travelers for fever symptoms (ibid). ITIS was tested by a team of researchers from the University of Otago, Dunedin, New Zealand, to measure front-of-face performance at airports. The scanners were found to detect fever moderately well, with an area under the receiver operating characteristic (ROC) curve of 0.86, which corresponds approximately to an accuracy level of 95% with confidence intervals 0.75–0.97 (ibid).

A new generation of screening is needed to speed up mass screening and improve fever detection accuracy. State-of-the-art ITIS technologies are often equipped with AI functions that automatically pinpoint each human face in a crowd and focus on just the right facial point for measuring body temperature. This not only saves time by filtering out the unwanted regions of the whole image but also can focus on and better analyze these small areas of interest (ibid).

2.2 *Surveillance*

Surveillance is a major step in controlling an outbreak [10]. The global spread of the COVID-19 outbreak is the result of human migration from one country to another or within a country. ML and language processing are two features of AI that have been recently used by the Canadian firm, BlueDot. In their AI-enabled approach, tracking, identification, and reporting of COVID-19 outbreaks was more efficient than the methods used by the WHO and the CDC. This result indicates the promise that AI holds and suggests that AI-based approaches can be used to predict the zoonotic infection risk to humans posed by climatic and human activity-related changes (ibid). In this regard, an approach that involves comprehensive analysis of personal, medical, behavioral, and social data obtained from social networking sites and other platforms can contribute to developing more accurate models to predict the health risk profile of an individual and provide suitable medical care. This approach, of course, raises concerns about privacy infringement,however, with a proper policy framework and safe AI technology design, such potential hazards can be greatly minimized (ibid).

While the authorities were waiting and monitoring the development of a potential outbreak from a small number of people who started to show symptoms of an unknown disease, these people would comment on social media to tell their circles of friends about their unwellness, and those people and their friends and relatives would use search engines like Google, Bing, and Baidu to seek information about the novel disease [5]. This collective behavior gave rise to surges of frequency in search keywords, which could be picked up by Web bots and Google Trend. Soon Web bots were scraping social blogs, tweets, opinions, and comments posted on social media, harvesting hints of illness-related sentiments and keywords right from the patients and their peers (ibid).

2.3 *Monitoring Treatment*

AI can build an intelligent platform for automatic monitoring and prediction of the spread of this virus [16]. A neural network can also be developed to extract the visual features of this disease, which would help in proper monitoring and treatment of affected individuals [14]. Such a system can provide day-to-day updates on patients and also provide solutions to be implemented in the COVID-19 pandemic [16].

2.4 Multi-purpose Platforms

Some AI platforms have multiple functions, and there are several ways in which such IoT platforms can contribute to combatting COVID-19 [8].

- Geofencing surveillance system: unfortunately, countries are facing problems with how to monitor many people who are in compulsory quarantine. As governments have already come to understand, not all people at risk are willing to comply. A simple electronic Bluetooth wristband could send signals about the person's whereabouts. Moreover, this could prove to be an excellent precautionary measure (ibid).
- Real-time alerts: the information collected at the airports about a passenger's health could be stored, and should any symptoms appear, it would be easy to see where the person had circulated. For instance, China was publishing each infected person's previous circulating area, such as bus lines or airports, so that others could react in time if they had been in the area and started feeling the mildest COVID-19 symptoms (ibid).
- Saving healthcare workers: a simple monitoring device could help immensely. Because medical staff are both exhausted and exposed, having a small, light wearable device that would monitor patients' biometric measurements (body temperature, oxygen saturation, heartbeat, and blood pressure) would help save time, and eventually lives, whether of the patient or the healthcare professional (ibid).

2.5 Treatments and Cures

Even long before the COVID-19 outbreak, AI was lauded for its potential to contribute to new drug discovery [3, 4, 13]. In the case of COVID-19, numerous research laboratories and data centers have already indicated that they are recruiting AI to search for treatments for and a vaccine against COVID-19 [9]. The hope is that AI can accelerate both the process of discovering new drugs and that of repurposing existing drugs. For example, Google's DeepMind, which is famous for its AlphaGo game-playing algorithm, has used AI to predict the structure of the proteins encoding the virus information, which could be useful in developing new drugs (ibid). However, as DeepMind makes clear on its Web site, "we emphasize that these structure predictions have not been experimentally verified…we can't be certain of the accuracy of the structures we are providing". Beck et al. [1] used ML to determine that an existing drug, atazanavir, could potentially be repurposed to treat COVID-19. In addition, Stebbing et al. [1], working with Benevolent AI, a UK AI startup, identified baricitinib, which is used to treat rheumatoid arthritis and myelofibrosis, as a potential treatment for COVID-19. It is unlikely that these treatments (particularly a vaccine) will be available soon, or at least to be of much use during the current pandemic. The reason is that the medical and scientific checks, trails, and controls that must be performed before these drugs will be approved, once they have been identified and screened, will take time, according to some estimates, up to 18 months for a vaccine [11]. See also Vanderslott et al. [1] for an explanation of the process that a potential anti-COVID-19 drug will have to go through.

2.6 Drug Development and Design

AI-enabled data analysis is being used for research and development of drugs and vaccines for COVID-19 [16]. AI can enable drug testing in real time, in contrast to conventional human-based processes that involve a huge amount of time. The time involved in the drug development process can be reduced significantly using an AI-based approach (ibid). AI can help to identify potential drugs for COVID-19 (ibid). The rate of vaccine and treatment development is much faster using AI than with the standard process. AI can also aid in clinical trials of potential vaccines and drugs.

3 Major AI-Driven Tools

To detect COVID-19, AI-driven tools are expected to have active learning-based cross-population train/test models.

3.1 Active Learning (AL)

As compared to passive learning (traditional ML classifiers), active learning (AL) is used to address a learning problem, where the learner has some role in determining what data it will be trained [12]. In an emergency (COVID-19), AL requires special attention so that data analysis and decision-making can be made consistently without waiting several days, months, and years for data collection. Again, exploiting real-time data (on the fly) is a must because one cannot wait for years to train machines and learn from them, nor is manual annotation and analysis possible (ibid). This means that instead of having a conventional set of training, validation, and test datasets, we need AI-driven tools that can learn over time without having complete knowledge about the data, which we call AL. In other words, the AL mechanism helps self-learning, i.e., incremental learning (IL) over time, in the presence of experts (if required) (ibid). The aim of IL is to iteratively help a model to learn to adapt to new data without forgetting its existing limited knowledge.

3.2 Cross-Population Train/Test AI-Driven Models

Beside the use of AL in ML, cross-population train/test models are a must in such scenarios because we do not have enough data from particular regions [12]. In other words, there is a need to automatically detect a virus in Italy from a model trained in Wuhan, China. For such a respiratory disease, it is essential to have cross-population train/test-based AI-driven models to make automated detection possible. In parallel, the collected data can be used to train models over time that are based on the decisions. Conventionally, in the literature, such a concept does not exist (ibid).

4 The Future of Artificial Intelligence (AI)

In the restricted business environment due to the global outbreak of COVID-19, AI can be used for consumer demand forecasting and supply-chain management. During lockdowns, Chatbots, which are AI-enabled auto-response algorithms, can assist customers around the clock. ML is going to be increasingly used in business. This may require significant improvement in the efficiency of algorithms used to moderate social media posts and visual content so that false negatives can be avoided, and reliable information is not blocked.

AI is efficient, fast, and reasonably accurate and can be used for long-term trend analysis. Errors related to human factors such as fatigue are not possible in AI. Hence, AI-based analysis is expected to make fewer errors. Furthermore, unlike humans, AI can be used to work continuously even under risky conditions. Factors limiting AI are higher cost, code limits, and machine dependency. With advances in technology, these limitations are becoming less and less significant.

5 Conclusions

AI can play a vital role in the early diagnosis and management of COVID-19. AI-enabled patient tracking is envisaged to be of great help in pandemic control. Appropriate and effective algorithms can be developed to enhance treatment consistency and clinical decision-making. AI can be used in different domains of COVID-19 such as medical, molecular, and epidemiological. AI can also rapidly analyze the huge amount of available data on COVID-19, fostering research activities on this topic. Finally, AI can be used to develop efficient treatment plans, large-scale prevention programs, and faster clinical trials on medicines and vaccines.

References

1. Beck B, Shin B, Choi Y, Park S, Kang K (2020) Predicting commercially available antiviral drugs that may act on the Novel Coronavirus (2019-nCoV), Wuhan, China through a drug-target interaction deep learning model. bioRxiv. https://doi.org/10.1101/2020.01.31.929547. Accessed 2 February 2020
2. Broad WJ (2020) A.I. versus the Coronavirus. The New York Times, 26 March 2020. https://www.nytimes.com
3. Coldeway D (2019) Molecule.one uses machine learning to make synthesizing new drugs a snap. TechCrunch, 3 October 2019
4. Fleming N (2018) Computer-calculated compounds: researchers are deploying artificial intelligence to discover drugs. Nature 557:S55–S57
5. Fong SJ, Dey N, Chaki J (2020) Artificial intelligence for Coronavirus outbreak. Springer, Singapore
6. Fong SJ, Dey N, Chaki J (2020b) AI-enabled technologies that fight the Coronavirus outbreak. In: Artificial intelligence for Coronavirus outbreak. Springer, Singapore
7. Hollister M (2020). AI can help with the COVID-19 crisis—but the right human input is key. World Economic Forum, 30 March 2020
8. Mudric M (2020) How AI and IoT can help fight COVID-19 pandemic, 28 April 2020
9. Naudé W (2020) Artificial Intelligence against COVID-19: an early review. https://www.iza.org/. Accessed 14 Apr 2020
10. Obeidat S (2020. How artificial intelligence is helping fight the COVID-19 pandemic. https://www.entrepreneur.com. Accesssed 14 Apr 2020
11. Regalado A (2020) A Coronavirus vaccine will take at least 18 months if it works at all. MIT Technology Review, 10 March 2020
12. Santosh (2020) AI-driven tools for coronavirus outbreak: need of active learning and cross-population train/test models on multitudinal/multimodal data. J Med Syst 44:93
13. Segler M, Preuss M, Waller M (2018) Planning chemical syntheses with deep neural networks and symbolic AI, Nature 555. https://www.nature.com. Accessed 16 Apr 2020
14. Stebbing J (2020) COVID-19: combining antiviral and anti-inflammatory treatments. The Lancet Inf. Dis. 20(4), 1 April 2020
15. Taulli T (2020) AI (Artificial Intelligence) companies that are combating the COVID-19 pandemic. Forbes, 28 March 2020
16. Vaishya R, Javaid M, Khan I, Haleem A (2020) Artificial Intelligence (AI) applications for COVID-19 pandemic. Diab Metab Synd: Clin Res Rev 14(4)
17. Vanderslott S, Pollard A, Thomas T (2020) Coronavirus vaccine: here are the steps it will need to go through during development. The Conversation, 30 March 2020

AI for Covid-19: Conduits for Public Health Surveillance

C. Unnithan, J. Hardy, and N. Lilley

Abstract The spread of SARS-Covid-19 virus has impacted the world as it continues to raise questions on the long-term impacts. With the absence of historic/big data sets, digital public health surveillance measures are informed via modelling using real-time data, which is collected and validated by public health agencies; and also aggregated/merged with self/open reported data by the public, via mobile apps and social media channels. This chapter informs on such conduits (using two case studies: Australia and Canada) that enabled AI-based solutions for informing public health strategies. Blue tooth technology used in contact tracing apps seems to allay privacy concerns to an extent, in both countries. Real-time streamed data collection to train predictive models and combining AI methods with active learning seems to be the way forward.

Keywords Public health · Nowcasting · Artificial intelligence · Covid-19 · Australia · Canada

1 Introduction

The SARS Covid-19 virus has pervaded the world in 2020 and has altered the passage of history, since it was first reported to the WHO country office in China, and was declared subsequently as a public health emergency of global concern [1]. In a short period of weeks, the impact of this pandemic led to lock-down of countries, travel restrictions, self-isolation periods and quarantine measures such as social distancing,

C. Unnithan (✉)
Public Health, Torrens University, Adelaide, Australia
e-mail: chandana.unnithan@laureate.edu.au

J. Hardy
Lifeguard Digital Health, Vancouver, Canada
e-mail: jeff@lifeguarddh.com

N. Lilley
BC Emergency Health Services, Provincial Health Services Authority, Vancouver, Canada
e-mail: Neil.Lilley@bcehs.ca

K. C. Santosh and A. Joshi (eds.), *COVID-19: Prediction, Decision-Making, and its Impacts*, Lecture Notes on Data Engineering and Communications Technologies 60, https://doi.org/10.1007/978-981-15-9682-7_2

as the world navigated a new standard of life. The pandemic befell a challenge for humanity as it has no precedent in recent history and no historic data available to inform predictive modelling or prevention measures.

For the discerning researchers and public health authorities, availability of real-time data, synthesised, curated and validated via WHO [2] was perhaps a starting point for tracking the disease. The data was streamed via live dashboards using geo-spatial techniques and provided contextualisation on global heat maps by research entities, such as the John Hopkins University [3]. Data sourced via these heat maps were adapted and used by different countries, for their public health surveillance.

However, concerns regarding privacy prevailed in many countries restricting the use of AI methods in predictive modelling. In this chapter, we discuss initial efforts in data modelling, utilising AI techniques and conduits for data aggregation that have been successful and an outlook for future methods as can be applied to Australia and Canada, considering the regulatory and privacy frameworks which do not easily allow for AI methods. The chapter is focused on public health responses and AI pathways in the 2 countries as it is being applied, in real time.

The main objective of this chapter is to discuss the applied methods being used successfully and conduits to data collection in real time (streamed) that is fundamental to the success of training predictive models using AI techniques, in the context of the 2 countries restricted by privacy regulations.

2 Data Modelling and Public Health Responses

In this section, we explain how the nascent data that was available was applied to modelling that informed public health responses, in Australia and Canada.

As SARS Covid-19 initially emerged, Australia had begun implementing public health preventive actions. First, it avowed a "human biosecurity emergency" under the *Biosecurity Act 2015*, on 18 March 2020 as reported by the Communicable Diseases Network Australia (CDNA) [4]. A high alert was issued as the Covid-19 virus feigned substantial health risks to the population that mandated immediate control procedures.

Moss et al. [5] reports that Australia had drawn on *clinical pathway models* that were developed over time in preparation for combatting influenza pandemics. The modelling was used to estimate healthcare necessities in the context of broader public health measures. An age and risk-stratified transmission model of the Covid-19 infection was used to simulate the pandemic, with parameters ranging from mirroring uncertainty in current estimates of transmissibility and severity; and overlaid with public health measures including isolation and quarantine of contacts, and broadly applied social distancing. Clinical expositions and patient movements through the health care system were simulated, including the expansion of available ICU capacity and alternative clinical assessment pathways [5]. Initial findings suggested that the pandemic would radically exceed the capacity of the health system, over a protracted period. Therefore, isolation and contact quarantines were rendered insufficient and social restrictions were mandated.

Accordingly, the Chief Medical Officer, various States and Territories, along with the federal government began issuing targeted, and legally enforceable steps with few distinct objectives [4]. The foremost was to swiftly identify, quarantine and manage infected people in the absence of an effective medicine or cure. This was followed by the identification, quarantine and informing contacts as there is no effective vaccine to immunize against the infection. Finally, strong efforts were being made to understand cluster spates and to manage them.

There was a fundamental objective to explain the epidemiology of Covid-19, so as to inform public health responses. These included the tracking of the virus over time, locations and people; diffusion dynamics; and categorizing special risk groups. There were requirements for testing and controlling community transmission of infection, localized to cities, regions or larger geographical areas with high density of population.

The total number of new infections; new contagions without recognized links to those infected, and outbreaks in impassable communities (E.g. residential aged care facilities, remote indigenous populations)—were prime considerations in public health prevention measures. These deliberations were evaluated against the capacity of health systems to respond to the virus, with tests, hospital facilities, availability of emergency front line responders and health workers.

Cases of Covid-19 and associated deaths are reported to the *National Notifiable Diseases Surveillance System (NNDSS)* [6]. The surveillance team has reported that reduction in international travel and domestic movements, social distancing measures together with public health actions have decelerated the spread of the virus, by 26 April, 2020 [7], in a report collated by public health agencies, emergency operations centers in state and territory health departments, public health labs and the Australian Government Department of Health.

In mid-April 2020, the Australian government announced the next phase of modelling the disease, using Australian data, to establish the current state of the pandemic, in a modelling method known as *Nowcasting* [8]. This modelling is based on real Australian data on the pandemic, forecast in 14 days, i.e. based on the last 14 days projected to the next 14 days. This method was originally developed by the London School of Hygiene and Tropical Medicine, based on observed hospitalisations and infections for 2 weeks. The need for real-time data using varied methods for such modelling is apparent.

In Canada, the federal government created the infrastructure to respond to Covid-19, in collaboration with provincial and territorial governments and international partners. The Public Health Agency of Canada [9] uses modelling to understand the progress of the country in terms of the pandemic. Models based on a range of scenarios are used, to guide public health action. Similar to Australia, the impact of measures such as physical distancing (aka social distancing), self-isolation, quarantine of contacts, and preventing ingress of infection from overseas were essential measures recommended by modelling. Measures to increase the number of health assets (such as ventilators) and human resources (workers), were also foremost in the measures taken.

According to Public Health Agency Canada, the modelling prior to the social distancing measures indicated that each infected person potentially could transmit the virus to 2.19 other people on average. As provinces and territories began their control measures and actioned public health strategies, variations emerged in the data due to differences in confirmation strategies and testing. For example, territories had low rate of infection transmissions. Canada also had a slower increase in total number of infections as community transmissions started much later when public health strategies were in place informed by approaches taken by other countries and their experiences.

There are 2 major approaches used to modelling in Canada namely, *Forecasting Models and Dynamic Models*. Forecasting uses a weekly approach using real data from the previous week, similar to the *Nowcasting* model used by Australia, except that it is undertaken weekly. Dynamic modelling uses scenarios created using a range of values such as average number of people an infected person may be in contact per day, percentage of identified and isolated infections, people who could be potentially in contact with an infection person—traced and isolated. Canada is at a different stage in the progress of the pandemic, as the transmission came in slower than other countries. At the end of April 2020, many of the provinces had shown levelling off the virus [10].

2.1 Public Health Surveillance and Artificial Intelligence

Primarily, public health surveillance is done from informed epidemiological data. The question that arises in a pandemic is how swiftly the data can be aggregated and used, and the role of AI comes into focus. Current research from CSIRO Data61 in Australia [11] synthesized some potential applications of AI in relation to public health. The protuberant among these applications was spate estimation.

As the use of mobile phone is surging across the world, the usage patterns are available with wireless operators. These datasets can be used by public health authorities to run AI logarithms to understand changing patterns of usage. And this learning can be used to estimate potential outbreaks. Learning from phone usage records of users, Machine Language (ML) is able to prototype and predict the bespoke assorted activities of users [12, 13]. If there are more people in isolation, the call volumes may also surge and these may occur at odd hours (early morning, very late night). There may also be decrease in call volume, which may correspond to deaths due to the infection.

An AI practice that offers much potential would be deep learning, which relies on deep data learning and high-performance model prediction [14] targeting to estimate accurate mobile application usage, i.e. anomalous calling behaviours and phone service inactivity. Public health agencies can estimate the potential size of an outbreak, near accurate, by applying machine learning and deep learning techniques.

When lockdown and social distancing measures are in place, AI can help analyse people's mobility patterns to estimate the locations where crowds are still gathering and specify certain geographic quarantine areas where infection can break out. With the mass population in most countries using smartphones and Internet, human mobility patterns can be estimated by using AI analytics based on geolocated, Twitter or other social media data records [15]. This solution potentially can trace the location of infected patients and track their movements, to predict the spread of this virus.

In embryonic literature, detecting temperature on human face, and breathing patterns have been touted as potential AI solutions in the pandemic [16, 17]. While potential symptoms of Covid-19 can be detected via face recognition capabilities of AI, enhancements using real-time data sets through deep learning techniques are proposed. For example, a dataset is trained to build an accurate masked face detection model, serves as a masked face recognition tool to check if the infected person is wearing a mask.

AI has been used for predictions in Canada. A new analytics dashboard from York University in Ontario draws on data from John Hopkins global Covid-19 map that publishes number of confirmed cases, and GitHub while using machine learning algorithms, database management programming language SQL and Microsoft Azure cloud computing predict how quickly the virus will spread across the cities and geography of Canada [18]. The tool is meant to assist policy makers to anticipate the spread, and based on this, make public health responses. The platform maps Covid-19 spread based on input by users, using answers regarding symptoms and travel histories to predict probable infections in an area.

Similarly, Flatten.ca [19] a Startup initiative from University of Toronto, is an online AI tool maps Covid-19 cases is designed to assist public health professionals project incoming patients and prepare allocated resources in hospitals. Interestingly, this initiative was triggered by the need of students forced out of their residences and work online for their research.

Bluedot [20] is a Canadian start-up company that detected coronavirus as it became a pandemic using AI algorithms to build prediction models even before it was identified in China. The company collects information via social media, government documents, healthcare data available freely, to build intelligence facilitated by natural language processing capabilities (NLP) and machine learning (ML). Every 15 min, it is able to track, locate, and conceptualise the spread of disease outbreaks.

3 Contact Tracing—The Next Mile

In Australia and Canada, the next wave of Covid-19, i.e. community transmissions was considered by public health agencies with contact tracing, as quarantine measures relaxed. Public health agencies usually assign a 'contact tracer' to interview confirmed infected people, who through scrupulous efforts, detects who may have been exposed to the person or have acquired the virus. Close contacts of a person may then be isolated, quarantined, or tested. Through this process, vulnerable groups or people with compromised immune systems may be protected in the future. However, in the case of Covid-19, this method is also increasingly challenging as it is labour intensive and requires tracers to use protective equipment. AI comes into focus here as countries begin to explore digital contact tracing apps.

Australia launched CovidSafe, a digital app for contact tracing based on a similar initiative in Singapore known as TraceTogether, which is available from Apple Store or Google Play Store, only via the Australian stores [21]. People who download the app are asked to provide a name, or a pseudonym, age, a mobile number and postcode. The method used is that whoever has downloaded the software will be notified if they have contact with another user who tests positive for coronavirus. This is enabled by blue-tooth technology and not using geospatial tracing. Using Bluetooth technology, the app exchanges a digital handshake with another user when they come within 1.5 m of each other, and then logs this contact and encrypts it. The data remains encrypted on a user's phone for 21 days, after which it is deleted if they have not been in contact with a confirmed case.

The application has two stages of consent: initially when users download the app so data can be collected, and secondly to release that data on their phone, in case they are diagnosed with the disease. If a person with the app tested positive to COVID-19 and provided their consent to sharing the information, it will be sent to a central server. From the server, state and territory health authorities can access it and start contacting other people who might have contracted coronavirus.

While the data is held by the government, only state-based public health authorities who are associated with contact tracing will be able to access this data. The legislation is currently being enacted to back up the assurance of privacy by the health minister [22]. According to the Australian government, no other agencies will be able to access this data, even with a warrant and court order cannot force the government to hand over the data. The registration data will remain on the government server until the end of the pandemic and then deleted.

Conversely, there was much debate on contact tracing apps in Canada [23]. Experts in privacy cautioned the deployment of such apps as the country has not been subject to the degree of surveillance by the government. A privacy witness seminar resulted in a policy brief that informed governments [24]. With reassurances from the privacy commissioner and subsequent validations, the Covid Alert, the exposure notification app was launched by Canada [25].

While the debate is ongoing, we considered other areas of concern and attention by the public health, that can be addressed with AI techniques. In Canada, social distancing/isolation measures were implemented, there was an added impact namely the Opioid Crisis. As people were locked in their homes or quarantined due to travel, the emergency departments in Canada, particularly in the province of BC, experienced a surge in the number of opioid-related cases. This added to the already overwhelmed health systems, which were already servicing the pandemic-related emergencies. At this crucial stage, the provincial government introduced the LifeguardApp [26] which connects directly with the emergency services using geofencing technology, limited to jurisdictions. In the long term, the project links into a mental health dashboard that uses AI techniques, to enable early warning signals at the onset of such pandemics, so that it does not become a twin crisis.

The global public health standard for preventing the spread of Covid-19 has been lockdowns, tracking infections, testing and social isolation measures. Very early in the pandemic evolution, Canadian organisations such as BlueDot has been able to use AI for early warning on potential outbreaks. Many other AI tools including mobile apps are emerging for early detection and contact tracing, so localised outbreaks can be minimised [27].

4 Conclusions

Covid-19 has been unprecedented and epoch based in modern history, as public health respondents navigate control and management of this pandemic. AI can no doubt be of significant assistance in managing the spread of the virus while implementing public health responses. However, AI thrives on the availability of current and big data to inform modelling for future.

In the early stages of the outbreak, Santosh [28] had pointed out that AI scientists must not wait for complete datasets to train, validate and test models. Rather, in parallel with experts in the field AI-driven tools must be implemented where active learning using multitudinal and multimodal data must be considered and AI-driven tools would be expected to work as cross-population train/test models. We are in conformance with this view as also applied in the 2 countries.

The methods and techniques as well as initiatives presented in this chapter are being applied in real-time, combining AI techniques of machine learning and deep learning to name a few. The chapter is limited to applications that inform public health responses, and *do not include* clinical interventions including testing, vaccines, drug discovery, etc., which are also areas where AI is applied significantly in both countries.

As the experiences from Australia and Canada have indicated, geo-spatial data collection via active and passive public health surveillance can inform early warning systems, while mobile apps enabled by bluetooth technology can assist with contact tracing, preserving privacy and not revealing individual geolocations. These conduits can be used to aggregate the data that is required to activate AI methods in training predictive models that can inform early warning signals and prevention strategies in public health.

Acknowledgements The authors wish to thank Fern Hardy and Madeleine Hardin from Lifeguard Digital Health team, Canada; and Nora Weber from Terracom Communications, Canada, for their valuable insights.

References

1. WHO (2020) Rolling updates on Coronavirus Disease (Covid-19), A summary, April 30th
2. WHO (2020) Coronavirus (Covid-19). https://covid19.who.int
3. John Hopkins University (2020) Maps Tracking global cases. https://coronavirus.jhu.edu/data
4. CDNA (2020) Coronavirus Disease 2019, National Guidelines for Public Units, Communicable Diseases Network Australia
5. Moss R, Wood J, Brown D, Shearer F, Black AJ, Cheng AC, McCaw JM, McVernon J (2020) Modelling the impact of COVID-19 in Australia to inform transmission reducing measures and health system preparedness, (Preprint)
6. NNDSS (2020) National Notifiable Diseases Surveillance System (NNDSS)
7. Australia (2020). Covid-19, http://www9.health.gov.au/cda/source/rpt_3.cfm
8. Communicable Diseases Intelligence (2020) Covid-19 Australia, Epidemiology Report 13, ISSN: 2209–6051. https://doi.org/10.33321/cdi.2020.44.35
9. Australian Government (2020) Modelling the current impact of Covid-19 in Australia. Available Online: Modelling Covid-19 Australia
10. Public Health Agency Canada (2020) Covid-19 in Canada, Using data and modelling to inform public health action, Technical Briefing for Canadians, April
11. Government of Canada (2020) Status Report. Covid-19 Status report
12. Nguyen DC, Ding M, Pathirana PM, Senaviratne S (2020) Blockchain and AI based solutions to combat coronavirus-like epidemics: CSIRO Data-61 report, Australia
13. Sarker IH (2019) Context-aware rule learning from smartphone data: survey, challenges and future directions. J Big Data 6(1):95
14. Sarker IH, Kayes A, Watters P (2019) Effectiveness analysis of machine learn ing classification models for predicting personalized context-aware smartphone usage. J Big Data 6(1):57
15. Shen J, Shafiq MO (2019) Learning mobile application usage-a deep learning approach. In: 18th IEEE international conference on machine learning and applications (iCMLA), pp 287–292
16. Twitter (2020) Use of Twitter social media activity as a proxy for human mobility to predict the spatiotemporal spread of 2019 novel coronavirus at global level. RTI Publication
17. Wang Z, Wang G, Huang B, Xiong Q, Hong H, Wu P, Yi K, Jiang N, Wang Y, Pei, Masked face recognition dataset and application. arXiv preprint arXiv:2003.09093 (2020)
18. Y. Wang, M. Hu, Q. Li, X.-P. Zhang, G. Zhai, and N. Yao, "Abnormal respir atory patterns classifier may contribute to large-scale screening of people in fected with covid-19 in an accurate and unobtrusive manner," arXiv preprint arXiv:2002.05534, 2020
19. York University (2020) Schulich develops analytics dashboard to predict spread of COVID-19. Research and Innovation News, Canada
20. Flatten.ca (2020). https://flatten.ca
21. Steig C (2020) How this Canadian startup spotted coronavirus before every one else knew about it, CNBC
22. Covidsafe Australia (2020). www.health.gov.au-covidsafe-app
23. Australia Government (2020) Biosecurity Determination. https://www.legislation.gov.au/Details/F2020L00480
24. Wells (2020) Invasion of privacy': Watchdogs concerned about apps tracking COVID-19 patients, National Post, the Canadian Press. May. Lemieux V (2020) Covid-19, technology and data privacy: a call to action for governments, PWAIS Witness Seminar, Blockchain@UBC. https://covidprivacy.pwias.ubc.ca/sites/covidprivacy.pwias.ubc.ca/files/documents/Policy%20Brief-4.0_FINAL.pdf
25. Covid Alert (2020) Canada's Exposure Notification App. https://www.canada.ca/en/public-health/services/diseases/coronavirus-disease-covid-19/covid-alert.html

26. Lifeguard Digital Health (2020). https://lifeguarddh.com/news-releases/new-lifeguard-app-launched-to-help-prevent-overdoses/
27. Greenwood R (2020) How AI could be pivotal in Australia's economic Recovery from Covid-19. IT Brief, Australia
28. Santosh KC (2020) AI-driven tools for coronavirus outbreak: need of active learning and cross-population train/test models on multitudinal/multimodal data. J Med Syst 44:93

A Pre-screening Approach for COVID-19 Testing Based on Belief Rule-Based Expert System

Tanvi Arora and Rituraj Soni

Abstract We are living in the digital era, where most of the hospitals in the developed nations are keeping the medical records of the patients and as a result, most of the traits of the COVID-19 infected individuals are present in the digital form. Based upon the data thus generated, which is present on various platforms over the internet. In this chapter, an effort has been made to propose an artificial intelligence-based self-testing technique that can predict the patients who should go for COVID-19 testing. This chapter presents a belief rule-based expert system to predict the likelihood of the person to be tested for COVID-19. The system thus generated can easily pre-screen humans without the intervention of any second individual. Based upon the classification results the individual can be further tested to firm the presence of COVID-19 infection. This method will be cost-effective, plus it will also result in inefficient utilization of the scarce resource of medical testing kits.

Keywords COVID-19 · Pre-screening · Testing · Symptoms · Belief rule-based expert system

1 Introduction

The COVID-19 pandemic has engulfed the whole world. The rate at which it is growing is exponential. Many researchers are working on finding out ways to curtail the ill effects of the infectious disease that has affected millions world over [1]. The medical practitioners are working day and night to treat infected patients. Although many countries are carrying out rapid tests to confirm the presence of the infection but

T. Arora (✉)
Department of Computer Science and Engineering, CGC College of Engineering Lancran, Mohali 140307, India
e-mail: tanviverma@rediffmail.com

R. Soni
Department of Computer Science and Engineering, Engineering College Bikaner, Bikaner, Rajasthan, India
e-mail: rituraj.soni@gmail.com

K. C. Santosh and A. Joshi (eds.), *COVID-19: Prediction, Decision-Making, and its Impacts*, Lecture Notes on Data Engineering and Communications Technologies 60, https://doi.org/10.1007/978-981-15-9682-7_3

still the number of available testing kits and the testing centers are limited, moreover they require the person to travel to either the medical facility where the test is to take place or the medical facility needs to be moved to the vicinity of the person who is to be tested [2]. In both cases, there will be human to human interaction, and this virus spreads from humans to humans. So there is a need to develop methods so that the least interaction takes place between the humans and only those individuals visit the testing centers who have been identified as the potential infection carriers.

The most widely used tests used for confirming COVID-19 are (1) swab test, which takes a swab to take the sample of the fluid in the nose or throat, (2) Nasal aspirate test is done by injecting a saline solution in the nose and then the sample is taken from the nose, (3) Tracheal aspirate test uses a bronchoscope that collects the sample from the lungs, (4) The blood tests are also being used to test the presence of the virus [3]. Although the sample collection methods are easier, the actual testing for the presence of the virus is quite tough. The testing modalities aim at finding the presence of the RNA of the virus in the cells of the infected individuals. The presence of the RNA is generally tested by using a reverse transcription-polymerase chain reaction [4]. Now if this process can detect the presence of the genetic material of the virus in the human cell, then the individual under investigation is said to be COIVD 19 positive. The test results are generally available within 1–3 days. Moreover, as per the current statistics available (as on 22nd April, 2020) on average, the countries have just tested 1.2% of their population [2]. This is because of the limited number of testing facilities concerning the population of the countries. So, there is a strong need to develop artificial intelligence-based testing modality that can pre-screen the potential patients, who should be tested for the SARS-CoV-2 virus [5], as if these virus carriers are left unattended, then the pandemic will further spread and may cause a threat to the life of many others.

Therefore, there is a strong need to pre-screen the individuals, before carrying out the test with the help of testing kits, that are limited in number, the artificial intelligence-based systems, can help to give an ideal solution for the pre-screening. To date, most of the work has been carried out to either develop a vaccine against the virus or to device the testing modalities based upon the blood samples or nasal swabs. But all the testing modalities require human intervention, which may lead to further spread of the infection.

In this chapter, we will be discussing an artificial intelligence-based testing modality, which is based upon the belief rule-based expert system, that every citizen can use and can check himself from the comfort of his home. If the artificial intelligence-based testing method suggests, that the individual needs to take the actual medical testing then only the individual should call the medical practitioners and get them self-tested. This pre-screening before the physical laboratory test is based upon the data that has been gathered from the existing COVID-19 positive patients. The motive of this approach is to test only the suspected positive cases, thereby this approach will help in the optimal utilization of the scarce resource of testing kits.

2 Related Works

Over the years researchers have used the machine learning models to predict the prognosis of the various diseases [6–8]. To combat the effects of COVID-19, researchers over the globe are contributing, by researching in varied fields like public health, prediction and possible tests. The researchers have mainly used the Chest X-ray images [9] or the CT images of the chest [10–13], as this virus mainly attacks the respiratory system of the humans. A research work titled Tools for Coronavirus Outbreak: Need of Active Learning and Cross-Population Train/Test Models on Multitudinal/Multimodal Data [14], has discussed the relevance of the Artificial Intelligence-based tools that can be used to fight against COVID-19 and they have urged that the AI tools are heavily dependent upon the data, so from the very beginning, the data should be collected systematically, so that informed decisions can be made if organized data is available and AI-based methods can help to work as cross-population train/test models. Artificial Intelligence for Coronavirus Outbreak [15] discusses the AI-assisted technologies in the fight against coronavirus. A binary classification model has been proposed based upon a neural network that is dependent upon the group method of data handling [16] using the parameters of temperature, humidity, density of the city, speed of the wind and the count of the positive cases per day were recorded for thirty days for the Hubei state of China where COVID-19 first emerged. They were able to conclude that the relative humidity and the highest temperature where the determinantal factors to prediction of the positive cased of COVID-19 patients. A Composite Monte-Carlo (CMC) based simulation for forecasting that has been augmented by deep learning-based network and fuzzy rule induction-based methods [17] to achieve improved stochastic perceptions about the further developments in the COVID-19, that can assist the decision-makers to make informed decisions. Since the disease has just emerged a few months back, the available amount of data is limited, the researchers have used an algorithm based upon polynomial neural network with corrective feedback (PNN + cf) [18], that can do forecasting with very good prediction accuracy, with the limited amount of data.

3 Materials and Methods

3.1 Signs and Symptoms

As per the statistics available for the persons that were hospitalized in Italy and deceased because of COVID-19, as of April 17, 2020, 76% of the patients had fever, 72% patients had Dyspnea, 38% patients had cough, 6% had diarrhea and 1% had hemoptysis.

Since this virus originated in China's Wuhan province [19], therefore one more attribute that makes an individual more prone to the COVID-19 infection is either the person visited Wuhan, or the person has traveled abroad, or have been in contact with a person who has traveled abroad or the person has any close contact with a COVID-19 positive patient. Each of the symptoms and signs can have three different values i.e. low, medium, high. Whereas attribute 7 and 8 can have values yes, no, or don't know [20].

4 Method

Currently, the persons are being tested for COVID-19 just based upon the suspension without backing by a standard reasoning mechanism. We intend to propose a belief rule-based expert system [21, 22] that simulates the physician's decision-making process, so that a uniform method may be followed for testing the individuals, so that the scarce resource of testing kits is not wasted. The statistics also show that the count of COVID-19 negative persons is also quite high.

The belief rule-based expert system generally comprises two apparatuses namely the database of knowledge and an inference engine [22]. The knowledge database consists of the knowledge that has been gained from the records of the COVID-19 positive patients, that knowledge may be uncertain and the inference engine is composed of input transformation, calculation of activation weights, belief degree update and inference using evidential reasoning [23, 24].

5 Prediction of COIVD-19 Using BRBES

The architecture, the knowledge database and the inference engine of the BRBES to predict the presence of COVID-19 infection based upon the symptoms and signs will be discussed in this section.

6 Architecture and Implementation of BRBES

The proposed belief based expert system will be implemented using a three-tier architecture [21]. The same is illustrated in Fig. 1. The top tier is the application layer which will be used by the user or the medical practitioner to enter the symptoms and the extent of the symptoms and to view the recommendation of the expert system. The second tier is the inference engine, which will contain the BRBES inference procedures and interact with the first tier and the third tier. The third tier will consist of the domain knowledge base.

Fig. 1 BRBES architecture

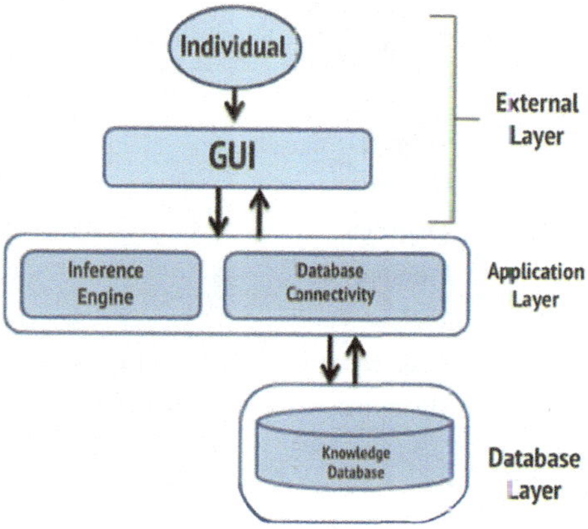

7 Representation of Knowledge Database

The knowledge database consists of the trees of the BRB, which has the antecedent and the consequent combination, the same has been represented in Fig. 2. In this, the root node represents the consequent and the leaf nodes of the tree are represented by the antecedents [25]. Now considering the symptoms and signs that are considered by the medical practitioners before recommending the individuals for undergoing testing for the COVID-19 as listed in Table 1. There are eight different attributes (the antecedent attributes) that are looked for in a potential COVID-19 suspect, and each attribute can have three different referential values, as listed in Table 1.

The rules are calculated using Eq. 1 where R is the number of rules, ki is the number of possible outcomes for each symptom, and N is the total number of symptoms. Based upon the Belief rule-based expert systems, considering the 8 symptoms and three corresponding values we are having 6561 rules.

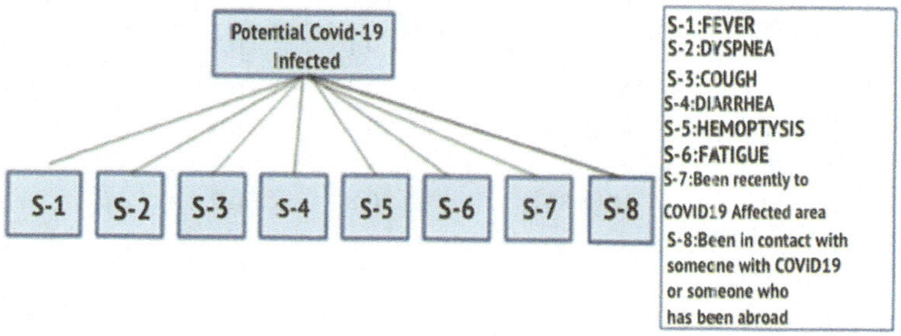

Fig. 2 BRB structure to predict the potential COVID-19 infected

Table 1 Symptoms and Signs

S.No	Symptom
S1	Fever
S2	Dyspnea
S3	Cough
S4	Diarrhea
S5	Hemoptysis
S6	Fatigue
S7	Been recently to COIVD-19 affected area
S8	Been in contact with someone with COVID-19 or someone who has been abroad

$$R = \prod_{i=1}^{N} (k_i) \tag{1}$$

The BRB is constructed by gathering the domain knowledge from the experts, the available data, and by using the pre-existing rules or by constructing the new rules arbitrarily if there is no past knowledge. For this study, the BRB has been developed using the expertise of the medical practitioners and the knowledge gained by the recent cases that have emerged over the globe. For this study, each of the rules has been assigned a weight of 1 and every attribute of the antecedent has also been allocated the weight of 1. Table 2 illustrates the BRB that is used for this study.

Table 2 Input transformation

S. No	Symptom	Symptom value (%)	High/Yes	Moderate/Don't Know	Low/No
S1	Fever	High 90	0.8	0.2	0
S2	Dyspnea	High 75	0.7	0.3	0
S3	Cough	High 60	0.6	0.2	0.1
S4	Diarrhea	Low 10	0	0.7	0.3
S5	Hemoptysis	Low 20	0.1	0.3	0.6
S6	Fatigue	Medium 45	0.3	0.6	0.1
S7	Visited COIVD-19 affected area	High 70	0.7	0.3	0
S8	Contact of COVID-19 positive	High 85	0.8	0.2	0

8 Interface to Gather Symptoms

The degree of the symptoms for the patient is collected by listing the set of eight symptoms and the severity of each of the symptom, by giving a predefined range of values namely low, moderate, high and for the symptom 7 and 8, the options are yes, no or don't know.

9 Results and Discussion

The symptoms associated with the medical conditions are generally reported with vagueness and uncertainty to the medical practitioners. Thus it becomes a challenge for the practitioners to precisely pinpoint the presence of the disease, therefore they recommend a set of diagnostic test's to firm the presence of the disease in the patients.

The belief rule-based expert systems can diagnose the disease when vague and uncertain information that is supplied by the patients. In this work, an effort has been made to analyze the test reports of 50 individuals who have been tested for the presence of COVID-19. For each tested individual 8 different symptoms have been recorded with the level of the symptom as low, medium, and high for symptoms 1–6 and yes, don't know and no for symptom 7–8 (Table 3).

The actual medical test results of the individuals are either positive or negative, and have been taken as the benchmark, to evaluate the correctness of the proposed BRBES system. If the test result is positive then the benchmark value is set to 1 and if the result is negative then the benchmark value has been set to 0. Table 4,

Table 3 A Sample snapshot of BRBES for COVID-19 Suspicion

Rule no	Rule weight	Antecedent								Consequent		
		If								Then		
		S1	S2	S3	S4	S5	S6	S7	S8	COVID-19 Suspicion		
										High	Medium	Low
1	1	H	H	H	H	L	H	L	H	1.0	0.0	0.0
2	1	L	H	H	H	H	L	L	L	0.1	0.6	0.3
3	1	H	L	L	L	H	L	L	H	1.0	0	0
4	1	M	H	L	L	L	L	L	M	0.6	0.3	0.1
5	1	H	M	M	L	L	M	L	H	1.0	0	0
6	1	M	H	M	M	L	H	L	H	1.0	0	0
7	1	L	L	H	H	M	L	H	L	0.1	0.6	0.1
8	1	L	H	H	M	H	L	L	H	0.8	0.2	0
9	1	H	L	M	L	L	M	L	L	0.4	0.4	0.2
10	1	M	M	M	H	L	L	L	M	0.3	0.4	0.3

Table 4 Suspicion of COVID-19 based upon BRBES & Expert Opinion

SNO	S1	S2	S3	S4	S5	S6	S7	S8	BRBES	Expert opinion	Benchmark
1	H	H	H	H	L	H	L	H	100	100	1
2	L	H	H	H	H	L	L	L	10	50	0
3	H	L	L	L	H	L	L	H	100	100	1
4	M	H	L	L	L	L	L	M	70	20	1
5	H	M	M	L	L	M	L	H	100	100	1
6	M	H	M	M	L	H	L	H	100	100	0
7	L	L	H	H	M	L	H	L	60	100	0
8	L	H	H	M	H	L	L	H	80	100	1
9	H	L	M	L	L	M	L	L	40	70	0
10	M	M	M	H	L	L	L	M	30	50	0

illustrated the sample symptoms of the 10 individuals who have been tested, column 2–9 represents the extent of the symptoms, column 10 represents the score assigned by the BRBEs system, column 11 represents the confidence level of the medical practitioner and column 12 represents the benchmark as identified by laboratory testing.

The proposed BRBES based system can search the rule base and can recommend the individuals for COVID-19 testing with 80% accuracy. The recommendation capability of the BRBES system can be attributed to the exhaustive rule base that is used with due diligence. Although the medical practitioners have more knowledge, experience, and intelligence as compared to this system, but the proposed system gives better recommendation as compared to the humans as it is not affected by the fatigue and biases which the individuals are prone and susceptible to.

The proposed system was able to give the correct recommendation to 40 out of the 50 suspected COVID-19 patients based upon the symptoms and the extent of the symptoms reported by the suspected individuals. It can be observed from Table 4, that the BRBES-based system is capable of getting better recommendations as compared to the manual decision making of the medical practitioners.

10 Conclusion

COVID-19 is spreading at a rapid rate, and there is a strong need to control it, which is only possible if the suspected individuals are identified and tested for the presence of the infection so that they don't further infect the others. The resources of testing kits are limited and the same testing kit cannot be used over and again. Therefore there is a strong need to develop a non-exhaustive pre-diagnostic test, that can be used time and again, by every individual, to rule out the possibility of COVID-19 infection or if the person is suspected to be infected, he should be tested to firm the presence of the infection. Therefore the Belief rule-based expert system, is the ideal solution, to encode the expert knowledge of the medical practitioners, so that each individual can get himself pre-tested at the comfort of his home and only the individual's that are suspected should go for lab testing for COVID-19, this system works with 80% accuracy. This system, will help in proper utilization of the limited resource of the testing kits and also save the time of the medical practitioners. The accuracy of the system can be further enhanced if the knowledge base of the system is augmented with more precise rules, after examining more patients.

References

1. Velavan TP, Meyer CG (2020) The COVID-19 epidemic. Tropical Medic Int Health
2. Cascella M, Rajnik M, Cuomo A, Dulebohn SC, Di Napoli R (2020) Features, evaluation and treatment coronavirus (COVID-19)
3. Kwon KT, Ko JH, Shin H, Sung M, Kim JY (2020) Drive-through screening center for COVID-19: A safe and efficient screening system against massive community outbreak. J Korean Med Sci
4. Rio DC (2014) Reverse transcription-polymerase chain reaction. Cold Spring Harb. Protoc
5. van Doremalen et al N (2020) Aerosol and surface stability of SARS-CoV-2 as compared with SARS-CoV-1. New England J Medic
6. Arora T, Dhir R (2020) Geometric feature-based classification of segmented human chromosomes. Int J Image Graph
7. Arora RD, Tanvi (2017) An automatic human chromosome metaspread image selection technique. Knowl Inf Syst 52(3):773–790
8. Arora T, Dhir R (2016) Correlation based feature selection and classification via regression of segmented chromosomes using geometric features. Med Biol Eng Comput 55:733–745
9. Wang J (2020) Procedures of health protection and control for COVID-19 during X-ray imaging examinations in Jiangsu province. Chinese J Radiol Med Prot
10. Ai T et al (2020) Correlation of Chest CT and RT-PCR testing in coronavirus disease 2019 (COVID-19) in China: a report of 1014 cases. Radiology
11. Bai HX et al (2020) Performance of radiologists in differentiating COVID-19 from viral pneumonia on chest CT. Radiology
12. Pan F et al (2020) Time course of lung changes on chest CT during recovery from 2019 Novel Coronavirus (COVID-19) Pneumonia. Radiology
13. Shen C et al (2020) Quantitative computed tomography analysis for stratifying the severity of Coronavirus Disease 2019. J Pharm Anal
14. Santosh KC (2020) AI-Driven tools for coronavirus outbreak: need of active learning and cross-population train/test models on multitudinal/multimodal data. J Med Syst
15. Fong J, Dey SJ, Chaki N (2020) Artificial intelligence for coronavirus outbreak. Springer
16. Pirouz B, Haghshenas SS, Haghshenas SS, Piro P (2020) Investigating a serious challenge in the sustainable development process: analysis of confirmed cases of COVID-19 (new type of Coronavirus) through a binary classification using artificial intelligence and regression analysis. Sustain. (United States)
17. Fong SJ, Li G, Dey N, Crespo RG, Herrera-Viedma E (2020) Composite Monte Carlo decision making under high uncertainty of novel coronavirus epidemic using hybridized deep learning and fuzzy rule induction. Appl Soft Comput J
18. Fong SJ, Li G, Dey N, Gonzalez-Crespo R, Herrera-Viedma E (2020) Finding an accurate early forecasting model from small dataset: a case of 2019-nCoV novel coronavirus outbreak. Int J Interact Multimed Artif Intell

19. Gong F et al (2020) China's local governments are combating COVID-19 with unprecedented responses—from a Wenzhou governance perspective. Front Medic
20. World Health Organization, "Q&A on coronaviruses (COVID-19)," Who. 2020
21. Hossain MS, Ahmed F, Fatema-Tuj-Johora, Andersson K (2017) A belief rule-based expert system to assess tuberculosis under uncertainty. J Med Syst
22. Hossain MS, Zander PO, Kamal MS, Chowdhury L (2015) Belief-rule-based expert systems for evaluation of e-government: A case study. Expert Syst
23. Yang JB, Liu J, Wang J, Sii HS, Wang HW (2006) Belief rule-base inference methodology using the evidential reasoning approach—RIMER. IEEE Trans Syst Man Cybern Part A Syst Hum
24. Xu DL et al (2007) Inference and learning methodology of belief-rule-based expert system for pipeline leak detection. Expert Syst Appl
25. Swartout WR (1985) Rule-based expert systems: the mycin experiments of the Stanford heuristic programming project. Artif Intell

Local Analytical System for Early Epidemic Detection

Yumnam Somananda Singh, Yumnam Kirani, and Yumnam Jayanta Singh

Abstract An Epidemic is a big threat to humanity. To reduce its catastrophic effect, many clinical practices and AI-based models are introduced to detect the onset of future Epidemic. An Analytical System can be useful for the prediction of an epidemic by collecting Quality data, modelling them and visualizing in different dimensions. This study deals with designing a Local Analytical System for early Epidemic detection in which the data related to human regular needs and responses are stored in the in-cube format. Analytical rules are used to produced faster pre-computed and pre-summarized inputs of the warehouse. Some desired inputs are selected from many local Warehouses which are then consolidated to form an incremental next higher-level data using the Layered Architecture style. This system can find the most commonly deviated data from the most frequently occurred patterns in the data submitted from the participating warehouses. The above-summarized patterns are mined using an FP-Growth algorithm to predict a new pattern. The patterns are ranked and inspected with their correlations for a possible unknown Epidemic.

Keywords Data warehouse · Expert system · Analytical processing · Healthcare system · Epidemic prediction

1 Introduction

A data warehouse (DW)-based healthcare system simplifies management of data and offers effective reporting with scalability options. It provides a consistent trust by

Y. S. Singh (✉)
Assam Don Bosco University, Guwahati, Assam, India
e-mail: ysomananda2015@gmail.com

Y. Kirani
CDAC, Silchar, Assam, India
e-mail: kirani.singh@gmail.com

Y. J. Singh
NIELIT, Guwahati, Assam, India
e-mail: yjayanta@nielit.gov.in

K. C. Santosh and A. Joshi (eds.), *COVID-19: Prediction, Decision-Making, and its Impacts*, Lecture Notes on Data Engineering and Communications Technologies 60, https://doi.org/10.1007/978-981-15-9682-7_4

linking across many data sources of the Healthcare system and other services made for the welfare of the citizen. WHO gives the protocol for Prevention and Control of the disease in which it is mentioned that nearly 50% of diseases are infectious [1]. To prevent infectious diseases, knowing the sources of diseases may help in detection and contention. Many factors assist in spreading the diseases, some are unpredictable, but factors such as season, climate, citizens' general habits, etc., are predictable. A study of the National Environmental Engineering Research Institute stated that COVID-19 has 85% correlation between temperature rise and cut in virus spread [2]. Many AI-empowered models are introduced to monitor and detect the future Epidemic by observing the data from many sources [3]. Besides the clinical practices, AI-driven tools are also explored for a better healthcare system. Many traditional methods need massive data to learn and have a long process to produce clean data. Active learning helps to learn within a selective target to generate a better result. It also supports incremental learning periodically in the presence of subject experts (on demand) [4]. Still, concerned agencies are unable to produce a suitable model.

This study deals with the development of a Local Analytical System for early Epidemic detection. Such a system requires good quality andmultidimensional data and quick learning. Many of such data are available inside a DW of most of the organized sectors across the globe. The system contains data mainly related to human regular needs and responses such as Citizen Health, Disease detail, Social habits, Tourism and Climate information, Health workers, their nature of the workload, Emergency data patterns, Insurance data and Service usages, sentimental data from Social media and Dashboards of the agencies, etc. The concept of the Fact table and Dimension tables are used to link between the summarized data (Facts) and the detailed data (Dimension). Many rules of Analytical processing are incorporated to give pre-computed and pre-summarized inputs to the DW. Usually, most of the data warehouse are standalone. For detection of an Epidemic, some selective parts of the Warehouse or data marts are interconnected and integrated using a Layered Architecture (LA) Style [5]. This Style facilitates easy access into many sub-data warehouse up to a certain degree following a hierarchical order and also supports incremental learning. Thus it has the facility to handle the multimodal data gather from the different warehouses.

In the proposed system, any single pattern or an item may not be the exact outlier, but collections of such patterns or items may become an outlier. This Analytical system helps in finding the most commonly deviated data from the most frequently occurred patterns among all participating DWs, or other data sources. It can analyze the data dynamically; it allows the data visualization in different views and zoom out data at different levels and also in different dimensions. The data from the above patterns are mined using a Frequent Pattern (FP) Growth algorithm to predict a new happening and drill-down up to the participating DW or the location to know the reason of the new patterns. The patterns or items are ranked and analyzed the correlations between them and their associated parameters to the sources. Such a new item can be an 'unknown Disease' that appears as a very frequently used 'item'.

2 Related Works

Many disease surveillance and modelling studies have been reported in [6, 7]. In 1993, WHO/UNICEF created GIS-enabled HealthMap for public health and many factors are identified. In [8], a Predictive Healthcare system utilizing data from many Health-care firms, Research organizations and Government agencies was suggested. Some studies used social media data for early prediction of disease [9, 10]. Earlier DW produced many final reports without any linking at granular levels of administration (District, State, Country, etc.). The Layered Architecture (LA) Style is suitable for a system that requires dependable operations [11]. This Style facilitates the DW to assign roles to the possible users. Many online analytical processing-based systems are presented to predict Disease outbreaks. Most of the earlier studies deal with a specific country or region [12]. Some study uses different types of available historical data from the health system [13]. In [14], a massive data is used in the study of Possible Dengue Outbreaks. In Finland, a disease surveillance system was developed using climate based factors like weather and air quality [15]. Many expert systems have been developed for self-treatment. Varieties of AI-based e-Health-care systems are also available for monitoring epidemiological data. It gives exciting dashboard information for visualization to help the healthcare executives in making active decision [16]. Most of the above systems produced a final output; however, it is difficult to link to different levels of administration (district, State, country, etc.). Giving some specific tasks to the participating user or data owners will be useful for quick processing and also controlling the situations at a local level.

3 The Setup Process of an Analytical System

Some theories of the setting up a Local DW (LDW) are taken from an earlier study [17]. Data are collected from different reliable sources such as extracted data from new or existing DW or MIS system. The data are stored in the Cube format for enabling modelling and viewing in many dimensions. A Dimension table is used to record the field level or detail data. A Fact Table contains the measured statistical data that helps in setting the relationships between its dimensions. A Star schema is proposed for the study, in which one Fact Table links to a number of Dimension tables. The benefit of multidimensional analytical processing is used to pre-compute and pre-summarize the data. The benefits of relational online analytical processing are included to analyze the data dynamically [18]. Two types of data are collected—(a) citizen-centric and (b) services. Many diseases are borne from water, air, food, etc. Majority of data are linked to human daily needs and responses. So, periodic data are collected data from possible sources.

Common consensuses are asked from all stockholders. The data are collected through different reliable sources by extracting from an existing local DW, MIS and Health care system. Random or unclean data are collected from Clinics, Departments,

Telephonic Interview, Social media, etc. Later, the stockholders are given certain ways to provide data. The unclean data are processed for cleaning. All contributions are recorded with high confidentiality. Many concepts of Extraction, Transformation and Loading (ETL) and designing a DW system are given in Oracle e-books [19]. During the extraction, the data are extracted from the sources. Transform defines a set of syntactic or semantic rules for extracting data. Other processes are performed to produce better Data Quality by fixing the misspellings, filling missing data, etc. During loading, data are loaded into the defined DW [20]. Many operations are executed inside the staging area before passing the data to a clean DW or data mart. Several Data marts are formed to gather similar types of data such as 'frequently occurred items', 'suddenly raised alerts', etc. The study follows a Star Schema in which one fact table refers to the different number of dimension tables. The dimension tables hold details on each instance of an entity concerned in the DW. Table 1 shows all possible lists of attributes of different dimension tables. There are several contributing parameters required for such study. However, this study aims to attract the most appropriate attributes from Quality Data Sources.

The Layered Architecture style is a development model that fits for a distributed system. The components with similar function are organized into similar layers and each layer performs a specific role within the system. The business logic used during the analysis is linked to these layers to enable quick changes in needs. It allows easy interaction between the different levels of data and can perform many analytical operations at desired layers. It also allows applications to reach down into groups of subtasks. Each layer can handle data in the hierarchical order as per a country's administrative system by enabling easy communication between the users at different layers. The user of different levels can do other operations at the same time (the concept of parallelism). The consolidated data from lower layers of a DW are used

Table 1 Description of the Dimension tables and their attribute

	Dimension Table	Possible attributes
1	Citizen Health	Number of birth, death, literary rate, diseases symptom
2	Disease detail	Disease name, sites, patterns days of rises and recovery,
3	Social, Insurance	Hygiene, Social habits, Cleanliness, Insurance types
4	Tourism, Climate	Visitors pattern, alert types, Climates, average patterns, etc.
5	User detail	User's unit, location, types of given data
6	Health workers	Types of Staffs, nature of duty, other details
7	Worker workload	Regular, overtime, extra duty, the pattern of overtime
8	Data History	new words, frequency, DW sites
9	Social media	New/medical terms, region/source of the topic, patterns
10	Service usages	Usage patterns of water, electricity, food items, mobile data
11	Emergency data	Types of an alert topic, pattern and source of the alert
12	Users feedback	Sensitive feedback, pattern and source of the feedback

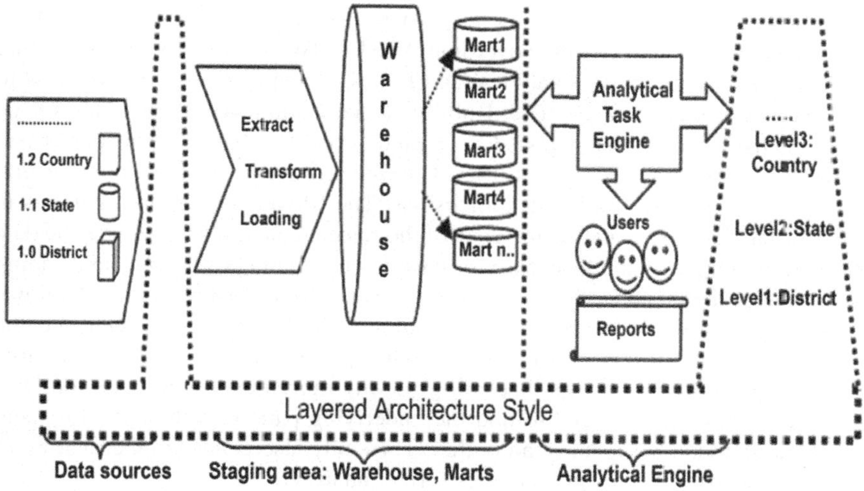

Fig. 1 Sample architecture of an analytical system

to generate the next higher and more meaningful patterns for allowing the Analytical Expert System to predict a new pattern.

The proposed architecture of the data warehouse based-Analytical system is shown as Fig. 1. It has many modules such as-(1) Data sources/collection units, (2) ETL process, (3) Warehouse/Data mart, (4) Integration module (layer style) and (5) Analytical Task operations. The selected data from other local warehouses are taken as data sources. Some of the local DW may be located in different locations. The corresponding ETL processes are performed. The marts are used to store some specific summarized data collected for analysis on certain criteria. Several Analytical methods give faster pre-computation on the cube data and also allow the data visualization in different views at different levels and dimensions. It enables dynamic analysis of the data and results. The dotted line shows the Layered style that helps to integrate all the modules and communicate among the users. It enables to assign different roles (extract data, analyze or apply security checklist) to the various users or data owners at different layers (community, district or State). Finally, the Analytical Task Engine enables different learnings, analysis and interpretation of the results. An authorized user can analyze report as per the requirement at a layer level or incremental way or a consolidated way.

4 Analytical Operations and the Findings

Many 'measures' are used to represent business requirements. The measures are the numerical values that represent a business metric during analytical operations performed on the Fact tables and their associated Dimensions. Example: AvgOvertime() to show the staff's average overtime. MaxUsedWord() to show the maximum used word etc. Some basic Analytical and Data Cube operations are developed to give interactive data analysis. The 'Roll-up' process summarized the detail of the data. It helps to zoom out stepwise for a prediction. The 'Drill-down' performed operations to examine the data at a level of upward detail. It helps to zoom into more in-depth data by altering its dimensions. The 'Pivoting operation' benefits in the cross-tabulation by rotating the view of the selected data. It summarizes the data enclosed in a lengthy list into a dense format allowing routine sort, count, and adding up, etc. The 'Slicing' and 'Dicing' processes are used to split a detail particular down into smaller parts that may help in more detailing. In a slice process, a detail specific is sliced into lower forms of data cubes. In dicing, the sliced cubes are once more decomposed into minor views that will give way more detailed information. The analytical operations are used to find the underlying pattern such as the Frequent Pattern of an unknown item, or an outlier. The study also considers the ranking of the items generated from the system for further analysis.

- Finding the Frequent pattern of an Item/event

The most frequently occurred items from all participating local DW are collected with the help of analytical operations. Then, the Frequent Patterns are mined using the FP-Growth algorithm [21]. It is scalable for mining desired patterns from the entire set of frequent patterns by fragment by fragment. The sensitive data are masked during the operations. In the example given in Table 2, three most frequently appeared patterns are COVID-19, SARS and AAAA. The item AAAA is unknown. The DW sites of each of the contributing patterns are recorded for further analysis.

- Ranking of events/words

Ranking algorithms give the rank of 'items' generated from the system [22]. In the example, 'AAAA' is a newly emerged item. It alerts the users to examine the concern sites 1, 2 and 5. Further analysis is performed by using the 'measures' established among the Fact Table and Dimension tables. More concern parameters such as the detail of Medical staff, their activities and patterns of usages of the daily services and duty routine, etc., are considered for better modelling, zooming, drilling down to the exact sources. Any deviated patterns may lead to abnormality in a site. Table

Table 2 Sample of Frequent Pattern

DWId/Site	Items
1	{COVID-19, SARS, AAAA, Nipah}
2	{COVID-19, SARS, AAAA, Dengue}
3	{COVID-19, SARS, Ebola, Zika}
4	{COVID-19, SARS, Ebola, Swine Flu}
5	{COVID-19, Avian, Mumps, AAAA}

Table 3 Example of the ranking of items/events

Words	MaxUsedWord	RANK
COVID-19	5	1
SARS	4	2
AAAA	3	3
Ebola	2	4

3 shows the ranks of the frequent items COVID-19, SARS and AAAA, respectively as 1,2,3.

- Correlation:

Several rules-based Adhoc operations are designed as a part of the Analytical Task Engine. Periodically, the correlations of the data marts are also computed. From the above findings, the correlations between most contributing parameters such as the usage patterns of daily services, overtime of the staff, climate, conditions (air, water, etc.) are analyzed across all contributing sites by visualizing the cube data in different views, levels and dimensions. Finally, the users of the concerned sites are alerted for the next actions.

5 Conclusions

A data warehouse-based Analytical System using the Layered Architecture Style is developed for early detection of an epidemic. Such system would be effective for early detection of an unknown epidemic as well, which is vital for taking up precautionary measures for contention and prevention of a disease from spreading further. The proposed system uses many analytical operations to give faster pre-computed and pre-summarized inputs. The layered style gives uninterrupted links between data of different levels, the user and their assigned tasks. It allows consolidation of the chosen data from numbers of local DW to form the next higher-level data. This LA style also enables incremental learning and can handle multimodal data. The Analytical procedures operate on cube data format, which allows the data visualization in different views at different levels and dimensions. This analytical system can find the most common deviated data from the most occur frequent patterns. The summarized patterns are further mined using an FP-Growth algorithm to predict the newer patterns. The patterns are ranked and inspect their correlations. This system enables to search for a specific source/parameter of the likelihood of a new Epidemic and make decisions for necessary preventive actions by the authority. However, the achievement of such a DW system depends on the confidence level of the participating agencies.

References

1. World Health Organization (2003) The protocol for the WHO study on the effectiveness of community-based programmes for NCD prevention and control. World Health Organization, Geneva
2. Study report (2020) https://www.neeri.res.in/ Accessed 29 April 2020
3. Fong SJ, Dey N, Chaki J (2021) AI-empowered data analytics for coronavirus epidemic monitoring and control. In: Artificial intelligence for coronavirus outbreak (pp 47–71). Springer, Singapore
4. Santosh KC (2020) AI-driven tools for coronavirus outbreak: the need for active learning and cross-population train/test models on multitudinal/multimodal data. J Med Syst 44(5):1–5
5. Shaw M, Clements P (1997) A field guide to boxology: Preliminary classification of architectural styles for software systems. In: Proceedings twenty-1st annual international computer software & applications conference (pp 6–13). IEEE
6. Bansal S, Chowell G, Simonsen L, Vespignani A, Viboud C (2016) Big data for infectious disease surveillance & modelling. J Infect Diseas 214(suppl_4):S375–S379
7. Greenwell F, Salentine S (2018) Health information system strengthening: standards and best practices for data sources. Measure Evalu Univ North Carolina, Chapel Hill, pp 58–63
8. Qureshi B (2014) Towards a digital ecosystem for predictive healthcare analytics. In: Proceedings of 6th international conference on management of emergent digital EcoSystems (pp 34–41)
9. Lee K, Agrawal A, Choudhary A (2013) Real-time disease surveillance using twitter data: demonstration on flu and cancer. In: Proceedings of the 19th ACM SIGKDD international conference on knowledge discovery & data mining (pp 1474–1477)
10. Myers MF, Rogers DJ, Cox J, Flahault A, Hay SI (2000) Forecasting disease risk for increased epidemic preparedness in public health. Adv Parasitol 47:309
11. Devi NS, Prabhakar L (2016) A data warehouse system for human resource management in a distributed S/W development. ADBU J Eng Technol 5(2)
12. Santos RJ, Bernardino J (2006) Global epidemiological outbreak surveillance system architecture. 10th international database engineering and applications symposium (pp 281–284). IEEE
13. Levin JE, Raman S (2005) Early detection of rotavirus gastrointestinal illness outbreaks by multiple data sources & detection algorithms at a pediatric health system. In: AMIA annual symposium proceedings american medical informatics association
14. Thawillarp S (2017) Evaluation of possible dengue outbreak detection methodologies for thailand, which one should be implemented? (Doctoral dissertation, Johns Hopkins University)
15. Heinonen G (2019) Data warehouse for the climate-based infectious disease surveillance system in Finland
16. Ziuziański P, Furmankiewicz M, Sołtysik-Piorunkiewicz A (2014) E-health artificial intelligence system implementation: a case study of knowledge management dashboard of epidemiological data in Poland. Int J Biol Biomed Eng 8:164–171
17. Singh YS, Singh YK, Devi NS, Singh YJ (2019) Easy designing steps of a local data warehouse for possible analytical data processing. ADBU J Eng Technol 8
18. Pedersen TB, Jensen CS (2001) Multidimensional database technology. Comput J, 40–46
19. Powell GJ (2011) Oracle data warehouse tuning for 10 g. Elsevier

20. Kimball R, Caserta J (2004) The Data warehouse ETL toolkit: practical techniques for extracting, cleaning, conforming, delivering. Wiley
21. Han J, Pei J, Yin Y (2000) Mining frequent patterns without candidate generation. ACM sigmod record 29(2):1–12
22. Brin S, Page L (1998) The anatomy of a large-scale hypertextual web search engine

Implementing Early Detection System for Covid-19 Using Anomaly Detection

Rishikesan Srikusan and Mugunthan Karunamoorthy

Abstract In December 2019, global communities were started to face a pandemic that was growing out of control. This chapter focus on implementing a system that uses anomaly detection on the data collected from geographically distributed subjects to mitigate the effect of Covid-19 disease by achieving the goal of early detection of the spreading. Other than the new diseases like Covid-19, most of the other known diseases and it's spreading has been already studied to some extent and have the vaccines and treatments. So new diseases like Covid-19's spreading can be differentiated from other disease patterns of transmission and can be seen as an anomaly. Also, as there is availability of wide range of smart devices, the anomaly detection can be a potential candidate for early detection and prevention system implementation for Covid-19-like infectious diseases. This kind of system can be used as an interactive tool to give advice and support for the end users. Analyzing the methodologies to achieve these goals will be the primary purpose of the chapter.

Keywords Covid-19 · Early outbreak detection · AI for healthcare · Anomaly detection · Pandemic

1 Introduction

Over the course of years, we are facing many more infectious diseases. Those are having its own properties. Due to its severity, some become epidemics, and some become pandemic as well. Later with our own immune systems response, intervention of medical treatments and vaccinations few may vanish from our environment and some of them become part of our society and occurs seasonally based on different regions and climates. We have faced Covid-19 pandemic late in December 2019. Due

R. Srikusan (✉)
AMIESL, The Institute of Engineers Sri Lanka, Colombo, Sri Lanka
e-mail: saririshi24@gmail.com

M. Karunamoorthy
Executive - RPA Developer at Ernest and Young, Colombo, Sri Lanka
e-mail: mugunthan45@gmail.com

K. C. Santosh and A. Joshi (eds.), *COVID-19: Prediction, Decision-Making, and its Impacts*, Lecture Notes on Data Engineering and Communications Technologies 60, https://doi.org/10.1007/978-981-15-9682-7_5

to the fact that we couldn't detect the disease earlier and stop the severity, which led our society into trouble, according to WHO [1] as per July 29 2020 16,341,920 cases were reported and 650,805 were deaths, which is a huge impact in the community and it is still growing. Also, there could be even more potentially dangerous infectious disease which may become pandemic like this. So there is a very clear need to implement early detection system for these kind of pandemics, which should be able to detect the formation of the disease and its nature of spreading among the communities at the very early stages.

As we are in the modern era of advanced AI technologies step by step accommodation of the AI in almost every field is widely happening. The goal of early detection of these kinds of outbreaks can also accommodate the AI techniques. Unlike the general AI problems, where we already have the data where the model needs to be trained on, here we don't have all the data which can be directly used to train the model. So to deal with such unexpected behaviors in the data, anomaly detection (AD) can be applied successfully. As this effort of implementing an early detection system can be possible only if we incorporate collective techniques. That is the purpose of the chapter. So this chapter focus on gaining factual knowledge from the infectious disease outbreak which is explained in Sect. 2 and the way of applying AD which is explained in Sect. 3. In Sect. 4, it is explained the implementation of earlier outbreak detection and the role it plays among the communities and in Sect. 5 the chapter concludes.

2 Learning from Outbreak

This section talks about the key concepts that need to be concentrated to implement a successful outbreak detection algorithms.

2.1 Key Concepts in the Area of Infectious Disease Outbreak

The studies on these immerging infectious diseases have been conducted at many levels and on broad range of scopes. Among those studies, there are plenty of them which can be useful in early detection of this kind of spreading.

Many researchers have studied the properties of the pathogen and the induced activity in the host body and the infectivity from one person to another. Infectivity profile of a person, where a person with an infection of certain disease the probability that he can spread that to another individual in a given day can be a very useful feature in identifying the nature of the spread.

Also one of the widely talked parameter called R stands for Reproduction Number is a measure which shows the average number of secondary cases getting infected due to a single infected person over his infectious period, should be estimated to better understand the effect of spreading inside the community.

Using the Infectivity profiles and the parameters R and all, if we can able to derive Expected Illness Incidents will be also equally useful in further analysis. Illness Incidents is a measure of the total number of infected persons identified with Influenza-like illness (ILI) at a given time.

The properties of the disease spreading can be sensed out by the measures and terms explained above as Infectivity Profile, Reproduction Number, and Expected Illness Incidents. Modeling of these terms from the available data will be a crucial step and will be an alarming status of the disease's spread and those will be discussed in Sect. 3.2.

2.2 Syndromic Measures Used for Early Detection

The clinical reports and data were only based on the cases that health care workers received, which may not correctly represent the actual situation of the disease spreading and also not a useful measure for early detection of these diseases. For the early detection purpose, the measures should be a representative of the case at an earlier stage. As suggested syndromic measures [2] are suitable for the early detection of this kind of infectious disease outbreaks. Syndromic measures are the indications that we can notice even before the laboratory conformation for any particular disease, which includes the behavioral patterns, symptoms, signs and so on.

As the syndromic measures the behavioral patterns like frequency of seeking health care facility, health-related web searches were used and the symptoms like the body temperature, other respiratory symptoms as cough, cold were also used. Among them, the body temperature readings will be a useful early detection feature [3] which can be measured through available smart devices globally.

Other than temperature and the stats that directly related to the disease, usage of data that are available publicly can also be better candidate for the early detection system [4]. Those would be using social media news feeds, travel details across the region like frequency of travelling to particular places which can be gathered from mobile apps, using these information, there is a strong possibility using an appropriate algorithm it can be identified if there are abnormal patterns in the data and which intern will be useful in detecting the outbreak earlier, also which can be argued that these data can at least be useful for detection of the place where the potential for the next outbreak, which is also a worthwhile attempt.

3 Anomaly Detection for Early Detection

This section discusses on the area of applications of AD for early detection of infectious disease.

3.1 Applicability of Anomaly Detection

We can see AD as the name suggests, it's, considering one as anomaly, if it is differ from what we expect to see. For example, if we expect a rotary machine to have a certain rpm and if it is different from what we expect then that would be an anomaly. By simply fixing a sensor to detect the machine's rpm will fairly be enough to have an AD system for any faulty operational conditions of the machine. Things aren't always simple in this way, there are situations where we can't say using one value or a range of values to compare with the current value and to detect an anomaly. Following scenario will explain this further through our targeted problem.

Let's think of the problem of outbreak detection which has the dynamics and characteristics as discussed in Sect. 2, where we have the required sensors which are to monitor the syndromic measurements from smart devices. The problem is how we are going to detect the readings as an outlier early as possible, using the measurements that we got. Here the issue is we don't have a certain value or a range of values to compare and quickly say whether the readings captured from the sensors are showing the outbreak pattern or not. The only thing we can say immediately is whether the individual sensor readings are anomalous or not and the anomalous sensor reading doesn't always should be the case due to an outbreak. For example, a person can become ill due to a normal seasonal fever. So the algorithm should be using some other techniques to detect the outbreak among the norm.

AD algorithms use models and forecasts from past data. For this to correctly work, the characteristic of the data should be unchanged over the time to the future, else there should be a somewhat accurate method to forecast the future trends. In an infectious disease outbreak, the later will be the case as the data always changes with changes in population size and the climate [5]. For better results, co-relation analysis can be used complementary to AD.

Also the usage of AD algorithm in this kind of outbreak detection can be made more accurate with the usage of active learning [6]. As the situation always changes with all the surrounding conditions the data that we are using to take the decision or build the model will change always, so active learning will incorporate the changes in the data and will learn over time.

3.2 Estimation of Useful Models for Anomaly Detection

As the basis for the AD, we should have somewhat accurate models and statistics derived from the data that is going to be inspected. In the case of infectious diseases as stated in Sect. 2.1, there were many studies conducted in the dynamics of outbreak which in turn resulted in deriving the required models and statistics to better show the nature of spreading and in turn will be useful in early detection of the diseases using AD

The study on Infectivity Profile [7] for an individual which was conducted based on influenza disease can be useful in determining the probability of the spread of such disease from one person to another in a given day from the day the 1st person got infected. To do so the parameter mean generation time can be used as the mean and the standard deviation to develop a distribution model which later will be useful in determining the Expected Illness Incidents.

Another study on the applicability of Infectivity profile [8] provide the relationalities (see Eqs. 1 and 2) which also a useful technique can be used in AD algorithm implementation.

$$R_t = \frac{E[I_t]}{\sum_{s=1}^{t} I_{t-s} W_s} \tag{1}$$

$$E[I_t] = R_t \sum_{s=1}^{t} I_{t-s} W_s \tag{2}$$

As shown in the equation (see Eq. 1) R_t denotes the Reproduction Number, I_{t-s} is the Illness incidents at time t–s, W_s will be the probability derived from the infectivity profile and $E[I_t]$ is the Expected Illness Incidents on current time t. The equations (see Eqs. 1 and 2) provides different usability from the same equality function. Given all the required values first provides the Reproduction Number and second provides the estimated Expected Illness Incidents. Both can be applicable in early detection of disease outbreak.

3.3 *Application of Anomaly Detection in Covid-19-Like Diseases*

Generally, AD is used to detect Covid-19-like disease outbreaks by comparing with expected or forecasted results from past data which mimics the region-specific seasonal infectious disease patterns.

It can be seen, how it has been showed in the study [9] conducted in all the counties in United States of America, using the parameters and statistical models defined in Sect. 3.2. Geographically distributed smart thermometer networks were used to predict somewhat accurately the effect of Covid-19 outbreak in one of the syndromic measures Illness Incidents levels. By using the Illness Incidents data prior to the pandemic period and the infectivity profile discussed in Sect. 3.2 and the equation (see Eq. 2) the Expected Illness Incidents were calculated for a certain period of time and which was compared with the calculated Influenza-like Illness Incidents using the current (during the Covid-19 outbreak) readings gathered from the distributed thermometers.

4 Detection System Implementation

This section talks about a system that consists of all the elements incorporated to acts as an early detection system.

4.1 Possible Practical System to Place in Action

As per Covid-19 studies, so far one of the succeeded model in early detection is the one used in [9]. Even though it was able to predict the impact on Illness Incidents abnormality, that model didn't use the spatial information, as that is what often provides much information in the case of infectious diseases. The spatial nature can be a better candidate [10] in improving the performance in this kind of early detection system. Also on the parameter usage, with the measurement of body temperature captured using smart devices, there can be other measures like incorporating other syndromic measures like condition of possible cough, cold and others by using voice detection systems or even by manual voluntary entry of such information can be useful in increasing the accuracy and decreasing the time it takes to detects the anomaly of a person's condition as having Influenza-like Illness, which will be a better approach than taking the decision using only the body temperature and wait for the temperature to stay for more period of time for the confirmation.

As stated in [11], a successful mobile app-based system can be implemented, which collects some user data, like their mental and physical status whether they have any kind of discomfort and their travel history and incorporating that information with the available data the system can find vulnerable persons and areas successfully.

4.2 Role of a Successful Early Detection System in the Community

Using the captured data and with possible AI techniques, implementing system which acts as a portal for health care workers, as well as to the general public in detecting the infectious disease outbreaks early and giving them a useful information, which guides the public and health care workers on the distribution of clusters or cases of the certain disease, may greatly help reducing further spread of the infection. With the use of web map-like feature with real-time indication of the risk factors will be a perfect solution for the early detection of infectious disease outbreak.

5 Conclusions

Advancement of AI knowledge gives us the ability to tackle many long-lasting issues in an effective manner, like that the early detection of infectious disease outbreak should be implemented with the use of AI. This chapter discussed the domains which need to be explored in order to implement such system and the possible way of using Anomaly detection and the possible practical implication which would impact the community in a useful way.

References

1. WHO Report, Coronavirus disease 2019 (COVID-19) Situation Report—190 Data as received by WHO from national authorities by 10:00 CEST, 28 July 2020
2. Mandl KD, Marc Overhage J, Wagner MM, Lober WB, Sebastiani P, Mostashari F, Pavlin JA, Gesteland PH, Treadwell T, Koski E, Hutwagner L, Buckeridge DL, Aller RD, Grannis S, implementing syndromic surveillance: a practical guide informed by the early experience
3. Bordonaro SF, McGillicuddy DC, Pompei F, Burmistrov D, Harding C, Sanchez LD, Human temperatures for syndromic surveillance in the emergency department: data from the autumn wave of the 2009 swine flu (H1N1) pandemic and a seasonal influenza outbreak
4. McCall B (2020) COVID-19 and artificial intelligence: protecting health-care workers and curbing the spread. Lancet Digital Health 2(4):e166–e167
5. Mehrotra KG, Mohan CK, Huang HM, Anomaly detection principles and algorithms. Springer
6. Santosh KC (2020) AI-driven tools for coronavirus outbreak: need of active learning and cross-population train/test models on multitudinal/multimodal data. J Med Syst 44:93
7. Carrat F, Vergu E, Ferguson NM, Lemaitre M, Cauchemez S, Leach S, Valleron A-J, time lines of infection and disease in human influenza: a review of volunteer challenge studies
8. Cori A, Ferguson NM, Fraser C, Cauchemez S, A new framework and software to estimate time-varying reproduction numbers during epidemics
9. Chamberlain SD, Singh I, Ariza C, Daitch A, Philips P, Dalziel BD, Real-time detection of COVID-19 epicenters within the United States using a network of smart thermometers
10. Kang D, Choi H, Kim J-H, Choi J, Spatial epidemic dynamics of the COVID-19 outbreak in China
11. Fong SJ, Dey N, Chaki J, Artificial Intelligence for Coronavirus Outbreak. Springer, Singapore

Covid-19 Classification Based on Gray-Level Co-occurrence Matrix and Support Vector Machine

Yihao Chen

Abstract Covid-19 is a new epidemic recently. Early diagnosis of related diseases relies on the analysis of the patient's clinical symptoms and kit testing. To identify this disease efficiently and automatically, we proposed an effective classification system by identifying CT images of chest based on Histogram Equalization (HE), Gray-Level Co-Occurrence Matrix (GLCM) and Support Vector Machine (SVM) algorithm. We collected 148 CT images of healthy people and 148 CT images of patients as our first-hand dataset, the size of which is 512*512*3. To enhance the features of the images, we center cropped the images to 400*400*3. GLCM is an efficient method to extract features focusing on the texture features and SVM can be accurately utilized to classify. In our experiment, we proposed a 10-fold Cross-Validation (CV) to ensure the reliability of experimental results. The results show that the average accuracy of our system is better than other common methods. The performance of our proposed method is effective for Covid-19 identification.

Keywords Covid-19 · Histogram equalization · Gray-Level Co-occurrence matrix · 10-fold Cross-Validation · Support vector machine

1 Introduction

Due to the emergence and widespread of a new coronavirus which was named COVID-19. As of May 20, 2020, more than 5.1 million people have been diagnosed worldwide, and more than 300 thousand people have died from the disease. The patient's early common symptoms are cough, fever, headache, etc. Symptoms of severe patients will appear muscle soreness, difficulty breathing, even death [1]. Clinically, the doctors diagnose the suspected cases through the patient's symptoms, CT images, and kit testing [2]. However, there are many asymptomatic patients who cannot be confirmed easily. Besides, the number of testing kits in some nations is limited, and some low-income people cannot afford the high cost. Therefore, it is

---

Y. Chen (✉)
School of Informatics, University of Leicester, Leicester LE1 7RH, UK
e-mail: yc306@le.ac.uk

K. C. Santosh and A. Joshi (eds.), *COVID-19: Prediction, Decision-Making, and its Impacts*, Lecture Notes on Data Engineering and Communications Technologies 60, https://doi.org/10.1007/978-981-15-9682-7_6

necessary to utilize the medical imaging for clinical diagnosis which is a low-cost tool and can be regarded as an additional diagnosis scheme, such as chest CT images [3]. However, a great number of CT images are not realistic for doctors to screen manually, and some less obvious features are difficult to be identified with the naked eye.

The machine learning technique has been developed significantly and applied in many fields. In recent years, the traditional machine learning methods are developing in the computer vision area by combining with medical imaging methods and the contribution of machine learning is raising dramatically. Chai proposed a segmentation system based on GLCM, Adaptive Crossed Reconstructed and k-mean Clustering to analyze hand bone CT images [4]. Reddy created a Brain and pancreatic tumor classification method based on the combination of GLCM and KNN [5]. Singh's research shows a credible result to classify Mammogram based on GLCM and random forest [6]. The researches above show GLCM can be utilized to extract CT image features effectively [7]. Dipayan proposed a Truncated inception net and the classification accuracy reached 99.96% [8].

Therefore, in this study, we proposed a classification system with high performance to solve the binary Covid-19 classification problem based on HE [9, 10], GLCM [11, 12] and SVM [13–15]. This system is built up to effectively classify the Covid-19 positive and negative images on our dataset, which can be applied in clinical diagnosis. The texture is an important image feature. Many research and applications are based on texture feature analysis, especially in medical image analysis. Histogram Equalization (HE) was applied to adjust the contrast and enhance the image features. Gray-Level Co-occurrence Matrix (GLCM) is a common method to extract texture features of images. And SVM is a good tool for the binary classification project. Our model has not been applied to classify Covild-19 image before.

Utilizing deep learning methods to classify CT images has a significant effect [16]. However, since our dataset is not large, some deep learning methods were not used, such as Convolutional Neural Networks (CNN) [17–21]. We may use CNN in our future after we collect sufficient images.

2 Dataset

In our research, we have taken chest CT images for 128 suspected cases, which are 65 ill cases and 63 healthy cases. To ensure the high quality of the images for our experiment, we selected 296 CT images totally as our dataset, which contain the complete lungs and are not blocked by debris. There are 148 images of the ill class and the rest of the healthy class, and the size of the images is 512*512*3, as shown in Fig. 1.

Due to the imaging characteristics of the CT camera, some labels which show the image dimension at the bottom and the curves below the lungs appear in the images. Thus, in the preprocessing step, we center cropped the raw images and the size of the

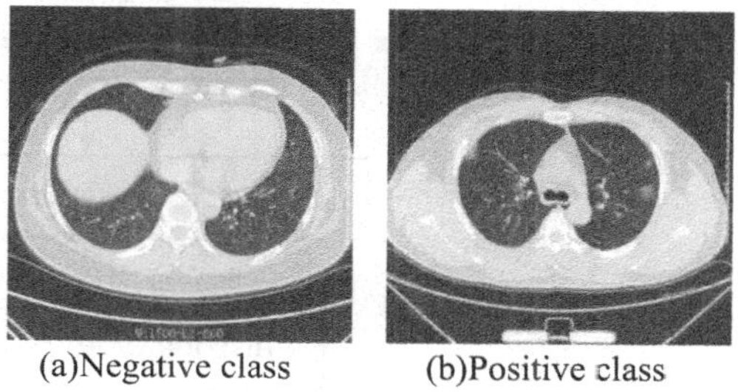

Fig. 1 Samples of negative class and positive class

cropped images is 400*400*3 to reduce adverse effects of the labels and the curves in the feature extraction process.

3 Methodology

With the development of machine learning and medical imaging methods, the combination of methods in different fields can contribute to medical image classification significantly [22, 23]. The contribution of our study is proposing a HE-GLCM-SVM classification system. Considering that the features in the raw image may not significant enough for feature extraction, we refer to the HE method to adjust the global contrast to enhance the image features. GLCM can transfer an image to a matrix and reserve the features in the matrix. The input of the SVM classifier is the feature maps with the labels. Thus, it is reliable to obtain classification indicators. The system flowchart is shown in Fig. 2.

3.1 Gray-Level Co-occurrence Matrix

GLCM is a classic feature extraction method, which represents the texture features of the images and is expressed as the connection between adjacent pixels. The main calculation steps are (1) gray image extraction, (2) gray level calculation, (3) calculation of the feature value between adjacent pixels, (4) output of the feature matrix [24]. By using this method, a large-size image can be represented as a small matrix, which can reduce the calculation complexity and promote efficiency [25].

The images can be scanned in four directions which are horizontal, vertical, two diagonal directions. To use the features as much as possible, we scanned the pictures in four directions and combined the four output matrices into an augmented matrix to be classified. The feature extraction process in one direction shows in Fig. 3.

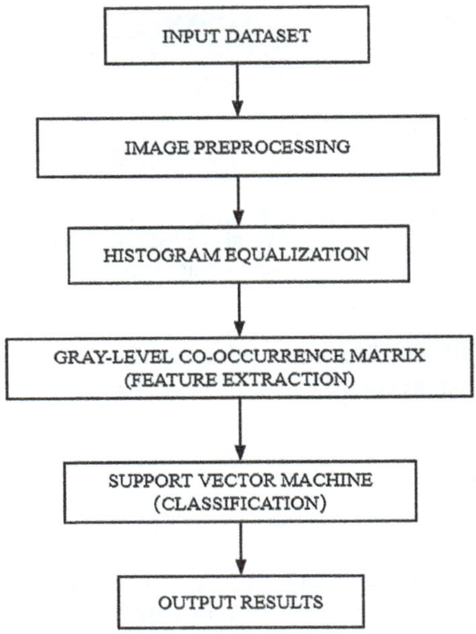

Fig. 2 The system flowchart

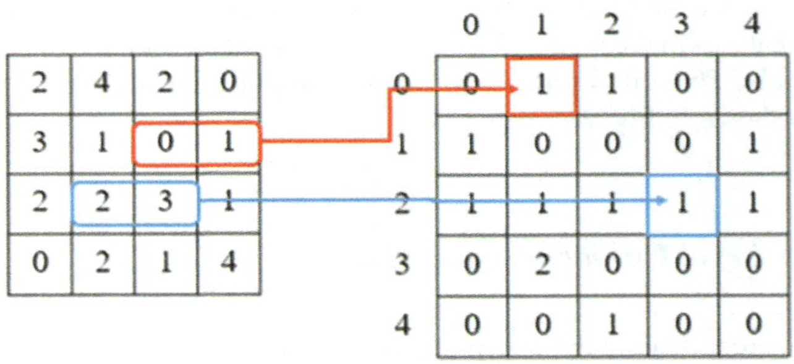

Fig. 3 A sample of GLCM in the horizontal direction

3.2 Support Vector Machine

SVM is a popular traditional classifier with high performance. The standard linear SVM is designed for binary classification problems [26–29], and it shows a good classification performance on a small dataset.

To train the linear SVM model, the "FITCSVM" function was utilized. Although our dataset is small, we proposed 10-fold Cross-Validation to ensure the objectivity and reliability of the experiment, and we repeated 10 times to obtain an average result. In our study, four evaluation indicators were used to objectively evaluate the classification performance, which is shown in Table 2.

4 Experiments and Results

This experiment ran via Image Processing Toolbox in MATLAB R2019b. The programs were run on the HP laptop with 2.30 GHz i5–8300H CPU, NVIDIA GeForce GTX 1050 Ti 4 GB GDDR5, 16 GB RAM, and Windows 10 operating system.

4.1 Data Acquisition

The raw images were center cropped from 512*512*3 to 400*400*3 to remove the labels and curves and put the lungs part in the middle of the images. We manually labelled every sample as "healthy" and "ill", respectively.

4.2 Histogram Equalization

To enhance the features of the CT images, we applied HE algorithm on both training set and testing set, since one typical character of the CT images is that the high contrast leads to indistinct features. Therefore, we preprocessed the dataset by adjusting the contrast. A comparison between the raw image and the processed images show in Fig. 4.

4.3 Feature Extraction

The images were scanned in four directions which are 0°, 45°, 90° and 135°. The size of the feature matrix extracted from each image is 9*9*4. To utilize the features in all directions, we transformed the matrix from the former size to 1*324. A feature matrix in 0° is shown in Table 1. Large feature values are on the main diagonal of the matrix.

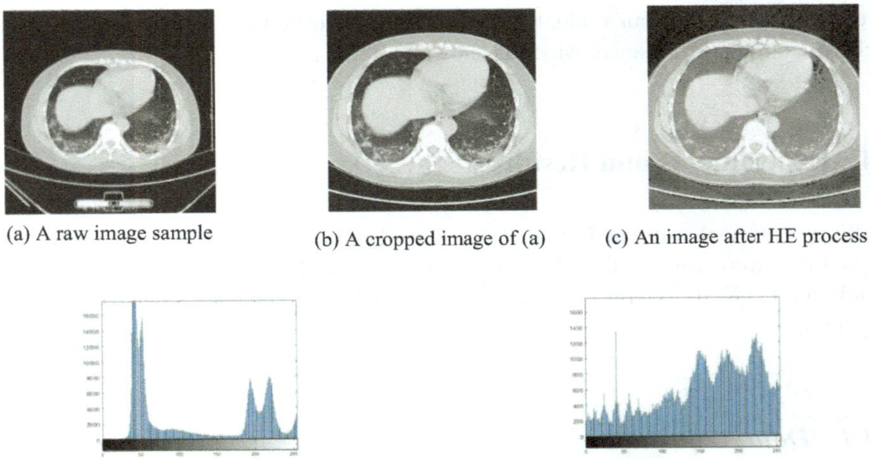

(a) A raw image sample (b) A cropped image of (a) (c) An image after HE process

(d) Histograms of (b) (e) Histograms of (c)

Fig. 4 A sample of HE

Table 1 A matrix in one scanning direction

3592	1576	378	135	31	1	0	0	0
1587	3080	1129	284	36	2	0	0	0
360	1141	4158	1477	246	16	0	0	0
142	247	1482	16309	4691	93	6	4	1
33	39	230	4652	13586	2483	558	124	100
4	4	14	113	2409	14445	4325	431	195
0	0	1	6	553	4284	11634	4608	1093
0	0	1	6	123	409	4637	16497	5949
0	0	0	3	133	200	1029	5952	16533

4.4 Classification

Four evaluation indicators which are Sensitivity, Specificity, Precision and Accuracy are used to evaluate the classification performance. The formulas show in following:

$$\text{Sensitivity} = TPR = \frac{TP}{TP + FN} \tag{1}$$

$$\text{Specificity} = TNR = \frac{TN}{TN + FP} \tag{2}$$

$$\text{Precision} = \frac{TP}{FP + TP} \tag{3}$$

Table 2 Results of our model and other classifiers

Model	Sensitivity (%)	Specificity (%)	Precision (%)	Accuracy (%)
HE-GLCM-SVM (ours)	71.95	79.23	77.31	75.69
HE-GLCM-KNN (ours)	61.50	76.93	74.86	69.63
HE-GLCM-NB (ours)	75.73	55.85	64.23	66.46

$$\text{Accuracy} = \frac{TP + TN}{TP + TN + FP + FN} \tag{4}$$

There are four main parameters which are TP (A ill class classified correctly), TN (A healthy class classified correctly), FP (A healthy class classified as an ill class) and FN (A ill class classified as a healthy class) [30, 31]. We ran the experiment 10 times and got the average results to ensure it is objective and stable. The results show in Table 2. Compared to the other two common classifiers which are KNN and Naive Bayes, the HE-GLCM-SVM model can classify the COVID-19 cases in higher performance. The results are in line with previous researches [32–35], which also show the superiority of SVM.

5 Conclusion

The aim of our study is to develop a high-performance COVID-19 classification system to help with clinical diagnosis. The dataset including 296 chest CT images collected by ourselves. Besides, we combined the HE, GLCM and SVM algorithm to solve this binary problem, which has great practical significance. The results show that our model can successfully help doctors to diagnose clinically as an additional tool. Moreover, we compared our model with other methods, ours shows an effective and reliable classification performance.

However, the results can be improved still, for instance, the accuracy is not high enough. In the future, more data need to be collected and we shall improve our model and other deep learning methods, such as CNN [36–38].

References

1. Xu Z et al (2020) Pathological findings of COVID-19 associated with acute respiratory distress syndrome. Lancet Respirat Medic 8(4):420–422
2. Fong SJ, Dey N, Chaki J, Artificial intelligence for coronavirus outbreak
3. Fang Y et al (2020) Sensitivity of chest CT for COVID-19: comparison to RT-PCR. Radiology, p 200432
4. Chai HY et al (2011) GLCM based adaptive crossed reconstructed (ACR) k-mean clustering hand bone segmentation. Book GLCM based adaptive crossed reconstructed (ACR) k-mean clustering hand bone segmentation, 192–197

5. Reddy DJ et al (2019) Brain and pancreatic tumor classification based on GLCM—k-NN approaches. In: International conference on intelligent computing and applications. Springer
6. Singh VP et al (2016) Mammogram classification using selected GLCM features and random forest classifier. Int J Comput Sci Inform Secur 14(6):82
7. Bernheim A et al (2020) Chest CT findings in coronavirus disease-19 (COVID-19): relationship to duration of infection. Radiology, 200463
8. Das D, Santosh K, Pal U (2020) Truncated inception net: COVID-19 outbreak screening using chest X-rays. Physical and engineering sciences in medicine, 1–11
9. Singh K et al (2016) Contrast enhancement via texture region based histogram equalization. J Modern Opt 63(15):1444–1450
10. Wu X (2016) Smart detection on abnormal breasts in digital mammography based on contrast-limited adaptive histogram equalization and chaotic adaptive real-coded biogeography-based optimization. Simulation 92(9):873–885
11. Sebastian V, Unnikrishnan A, Balakrishnan K (2012) Gray level co-occurrence matrices: generalisation and some new features. arXiv preprint arXiv:1205.4831
12. Li W (2020) Gingivitis identification via multichannel gray-level co-occurrence matrix and particle swarm optimization neural network. Int J Imaging Syst Technol 30(2):401–411
13. Suykens JA, Vandewalle J (1999) Least squares support vector machine classifiers. Neural Process Lett 9(3):293–300
14. Li Y (2017) Detection of dendritic spines using wavelet packet entropy and fuzzy support vector machine. CNS & Neurological Disorders—Drug Targets 16(2):116–121
15. Lu HM (2016) Facial emotion recognition based on biorthogonal wavelet entropy, fuzzy support vector machine, and stratified cross validation. IEEE Access 4:8375–8385
16. Li L et al (2020) Artificial intelligence distinguishes COVID-19 from community acquired pneumonia on chest CT. Radiology, 200905
17. Jiang X (2020) Fingerspelling identification for Chinese sign language via AlexNet-based transfer learning and Adam optimizer. Scient Programm, 2020
18. Jiang X, Chang L (2020) Classification of Alzheimer's disease via eight-layer convolutional neural network with batch normalization and dropout techniques. J Med Imaging Health Inform 10(5):1040–1048
19. Chen Y (2020) Cerebral micro-bleeding identification based on a nine-layer convolutional neural network with stochastic pooling. Concurr Comput: Practice Exp 31(1):e5130
20. Sangaiah AK (2020) Alcoholism identification via convolutional neural network based on parametric ReLU, dropout, and batch normalization. Neural Comput Appl 32:665–680
21. Govindaraj VV (2019) High performance multiple sclerosis classification by data augmentation and AlexNet transfer learning model. J Med Imaging Health Inform 9(9):2012–2021
22. De Bruijne M (2016) Machine learning approaches in medical image analysis: From detection to diagnosis. Elsevier
23. Nanni L, Lumini A, Brahnam S (2010) Local binary patterns variants as texture descriptors for medical image analysis. Artif Intelligence Med 49(2):117–125
24. Hua B, Fu-Long M, Li-Cheng J (2006) Research on computation of GLCM of image texture. Acta Electronica Sinica 1(1):155–158
25. Kekre H et al (2010) Image Retrieval using Texture Features extracted from GLCM, LBG and KPE. Int J Comput Theory Eng 2(5):695
26. Gorriz JM, Ramírez J (2016) Wavelet entropy and directed acyclic graph support vector machine for detection of patients with unilateral hearing loss in MRI scanning. Front Comput Neurosc 10
27. Zhou X-X (2016) Comparison of machine learning methods for stationary wavelet entropy-based multiple sclerosis detection: decision tree, k-nearest neighbors, and support vector machine. Simulation 92(9):861–871
28. Chen M (2016) Morphological analysis of dendrites and spines by hybridization of ridge detection with twin support vector machine. PeerJ 4
29. Yang M (2016) dual-tree complex wavelet transform and twin support vector machine for pathological brain detection. Appl Sci 6(6)

30. Koestinger M et al (2012) Large scale metric learning from equivalence constraints. In: 2012 IEEE conference on computer vision and pattern recognition. IEEE
31. Veropoulos K, Campbell C, Cristianini N (1999) Controlling the sensitivity of support vector machines. In: Proceedings of the international joint conference on AI
32. Liu G, Pathological brain detection in MRI scanning by wavelet packet Tsallis entropy and fuzzy support vector machine. SpringerPlus 4(1)
33. Chen S, Yang J-F, Phillips P (2015) Magnetic resonance brain image classification based on weighted-type fractional Fourier transform and nonparallel support vector machine. Int J Imaging Syst Technol 25(4):317–327
34. Yang J (2015) Identification of green, Oolong and black teas in China via wavelet packet entropy and fuzzy support vector machine. Entropy 17(10):6663–6682
35. Liu A (2015) Magnetic resonance brain image classification via stationary wavelet transform and generalized eigenvalue proximal support vector machine. J Med Imaging Health Inform 5(7):1395–1403
36. Jiang X (2019) Chinese Sign language fingerspelling recognition via six-layer convolutional neural network with leaky rectified linear units for therapy and rehabilitation. J Med Imaging Health Inform 9(9):2031–2038
37. Tang C (2019) Cerebral micro-bleeding detection based on densely connected neural network. Front Neurosci 13
38. Xie S (2019) Alcoholism identification based on an AlexNet transfer learning model. Front Psychiatry 10

Rough Sets in COVID-19 to Predict Symptomatic Cases

Haribhau R. Bhapkar, Parikshit N. Mahalle, Gitanjali R. Shinde, and Mufti Mahmud

Abstract Rough set theory is a new mathematical or set-theoretical practice to study inadequate knowledge. There are many use cases in the real world where there is a lack of crisp knowledge. In view of this, many Scientists have been attempted to address anomalies associated with imperfect knowledge for a long time. In recent times, computer and mathematics researchers have been trying to resolve this decisive issue, mainly in artificial intelligence province. The COVID-19 pandemic encroaches the harmony of the whole world. Many patients of COVID-19 have different symptoms, so it is very difficult to carry out the symptoms-based prediction COVID-19. However, the rough set theory approach help to minimize the number of attributes from the underlined decision table. This work defines the decision table having patients and symptoms of the COVID-19 in the rows and columns respectively. By studying data indiscernibility, elementary sets are specified for each attribute. Moreover, lower approximation, upper approximation, class of rough sets and accuracy of approximation are defined for different individual or group symptoms. This proposed work investigates whether particular symptoms belong to the decision set or not and

H. R. Bhapkar
MIT School of Engineering, Department of Mathematics, MIT ADT University's, Pune, Maharashtra, India
e-mail: hrbhapkar@gmail.com

P. N. Mahalle · G. R. Shinde (✉)
Department of Computer Engineering, Smt. Kashibai Navale College of Engineering, Pune, Maharashtra, India
e-mail: gr83gita@gmail.com

P. N. Mahalle
e-mail: aalborg.pnm@gmail.com

P. N. Mahalle
Department of Communication, Media and Information Technologies, Aalborg University, Copenhagen, Denmark

M. Mahmud
Department of Computing and Technology, Nottingham Trent University, Clifton, Nottingham NG11 8NS, UK
e-mail: mufti.mahmud@ntu.ac.uk

K. C. Santosh and A. Joshi (eds.), *COVID-19: Prediction, Decision-Making, and its Impacts*, Lecture Notes on Data Engineering and Communications Technologies 60, https://doi.org/10.1007/978-981-15-9682-7_7

also the accuracy of observations is calculated and analyzed. The probability of having COVID-19 is defined by considering the different sets of attributes. The main objective of this work is to minimize the number of symptoms of COVID-19 by rough set theory approach for better decision making. This symptoms-based prediction could help us while checking patients and decision-makers could be benefited while making policies and guidelines.

Keywords COVID-19 · Rough set · Indiscernibility · Prediction

1 Introduction

The origin of coronavirus is found in china dated December 2019. This virus severely affects the respiratory system of humans. In the duration of merely just three months COVID-19 has become a pandemic faced by 213 countries around the world. So far 5.5 million people are infected with the disease [1]. The death count has reached a total of 353334. This virus is contagious and it is spreading in the form of droplets. The symptoms of COVID-19 have been in the range of mild to very severe. In very severe cases it is extending to death in a short time of two to three weeks. After the patient has been exposed to the virus, the symptoms can be experienced by the patient in the duration of 2–14 days. The symptoms typically include fever, cough, shortness of breath and pneumonia [2]. In such a pandemic situation efficient emergency management system is required with available data and technology in order to improve the management of this pandemic situation. Trending new cutting-edge technologies are trying to create out current emergency management systems more efficient and intelligent. For an extended period of time, there was a struggle to combine technology with the disaster response process. But available new technologies have found a better path for this integration. Domains like artificial intelligence (AI), the Internet of things and blockchain technology are providing a solution to deal with real-time sensitive data so that it can be effectively useful in the decision-making process.

Tremendous work has been going on analysis, forecasting and prediction of COVID-19 spread rate. Fast and efficient predictions are required in such a pandemic situation to reduce the spared rate of the disease. Various models and approaches are proposed by researchers for analysis and prediction of COVID-19 [3–5] i.e. differential equations, SIR (Suspect Infected Recovered) and extended SIR models, Machine learning, deep learning approaches, etc. [6–8]. Every model and approach have its own pros and cons. The efficiency and correctness of models and approaches are based on data and parameters used for analysis. Hence it might possible that a particular model is beneficial in certain conditions only. Traditional mathematical models are good for estimations and machine learning/deep learning approaches are best suited when big data is available for training the model.

Roda et al. [9] presented a comparison of the SIR and SEIR model with confirmed case data of Wuhan city. This data is taken after lockdown hence isolation and quarantine plays are a major role in this prediction. Huang et al. [10] presents the logistic model and shows that infection of COVID-19 is spatially dependent. Bhattacharjee et al. [11] present the effect of environmental factors on the spread rate of COVID-19, in this study parameters like temperature, wind speed and humidity are considered for analysis. Study shows that there is not any specific impact environmental factor on the spread rate. Dowd et al. [12] presented the impact of age and gender on the spread rate of COVID-19, the results of the study show that coronavirus effects more on elder people. In the literature, researchers have taken datasets from various sources World Health Organization (WHO), the Chinese Center for Disease Control and Prevention, Johns Hopkins University, newspaper sites, Github repositories and also from social media. In the literature, various parameters are considered like social parameters (i.e. awareness, social distancing, government policies, mobility, availability of medical facilities, a period of quarantine and isolation), Metrological parameters (i.e. temperature, wind speed, humidity, geographical location), COVID-19 specific parameters (i.e. daily death count, infection rate, incubation period) and patient-specific parameters (i.e. age, gender, underline diseases) [4]. There is a need of an approach that can make predictions whether a person has an infection of COVID-19 based on symptoms.

In a pandemic situation like CVOID-19 available information may be vague and imperfect. Rough set theory is one of the approaches that can be used with such data for the prediction of COVID-19. In this work, an application rough theory approach is proposed for predictions of COVID-19.

Rough set theory is a new mathematical or set-theoretical approach to study imperfect knowledge. Many mathematicians, logicians and philosophers have been attempted to address anomalies associated with imperfect knowledge for a long time. In recent times, computer researchers have been trying to resolve this decisive issue, mainly in AI province. To cognize and manipulate imperfect information, there are many approaches. One of them is the Fuzzy sets and the other attempt is the rough set theory approach. Rough set theory approach is perceived to be of major significance to decision analysis, pattern recognition, expert systems, machine learning, knowledge acquisitions and many more [13–20]. It is developed as the independent branch of mathematics as it does not require any more crisp information regarding the data. Practically, almost all the concepts we are studying and using in the usual language are vague. This is the reason for the importance of vagueness to philosophers and scientists. It is generally associated with the boundary region approach. Rough set theory is defined quite usually by using interior, closure and boundary approximations [21]. The main contributions of this paper are the study of existing approaches used for predictions and their limitations, application of rough set theory for COVID-19 prediction, building mathematical formulations by eliminating non-important attributes from decision table for better predictions.

2 Preliminaries

2.1 Rough Sets

In this work, the rough set theory approach is used to enhance the symptom-based prediction of COVID-19. The theoretical perspective of this to develop a symptoms-based model of COVID-19 is given below.

A relation which is reflexive, symmetric and transitive is called an equivalence relation.

Let U be the universal set and A be non-empty finite set of attributes. Therefore, S = (U, A) is an information system, Let P $\subseteq$ A and a is in A, An Indiscernibility relation is defined as **Ind$_S$ (P)** = {(u, v)/(u) = (v), for all aP}

A Relation R_* (X) is called the R-Lower approximation of set X with respect to R if R_* (X) = {x/R(x) $\subseteq$ X}.

It is called R- upper approximation if R^* (X) = {x/R(x) $\cap$ X $\neq \emptyset$}.

A boundary region is given by B_R (X) = R^* (X)−R_* (X).

Let B $\subseteq$ A, C $\subseteq$ A, a set of attributes C depends on B, if all values of attributes from C are uniquely governed by values of attributes from B. Alternately, C depends totally on B, if there exists a functional dependency relation between values of C and B.

2.2 COVID-19

By considering all aspects, it is found that the most mutual symptoms among so many patients who were quarantined or hospitalized due to COVID-19 are as follows.

Fever: 99%, Fatigue: 70%, A dry cough: 59%, Loss of appetite: 40%, Body aches: 35%, Shortness of breath: 31%, Mucus or phlegm: 27% [14].

Further symptoms may consist of headache, sore throat, chills, sometimes with shaking, loss of smell or taste, stuffy nose, vomiting or nausea, diarrhea. For the sake of minimalism, we first explain this approach intuitively. Data are habitually presented in the form of a table, columns are labeled by attributes, rows by entities of interest and entries of the table are attribute values. In this work, Table 1 comprises information about patients suffering from COVID-19. (Strictly talking about their ID's). Attributes can be Fever, Fatigue, A dry cough, Loss of appetite, body aches, shortness of breath, Mucus, etc. Such tables are known as information systems of COVID-19, or information tables, or attribute-value tables. Consider the following information table (Table 1) of COVID-19. Suppose we have data of 10 patients, which is shown in Table 1. Columns of the table of COVID-19 (COVID-19 table) are labeled by attributes (symptoms) as well as rows are labeled by patients. However, entries of the COVID-19 table are attribute values. Therefore, each row of the table epitomizes all information about the corresponding patient.

Table 1 COVID-19 symptoms analysis

Patients	Fever	A dry cough	Body aches	Loss of appetite	Shortness of breath	Fatigue	Mucus	Stuffy nose	Nausea	COVID-19
P_1	H	Yes	No	No	Yes	Yes	No	Yes	No	Yes
P_2	H	No	Yes	Yes	Yes	No	Yes	No	Yes	No
P_3	H	Yes	Yes	Yes	Yes	Yes	Yes	No	Yes	Yes
P_4	H	Yes	Yes	No	No	Yes	No	Yes	No	Yes
P_5	N	Yes	Yes	Yes	No	No	Yes	No	Yes	No
P_6	H	No	Yes	No	No	Yes	No	Yes	Yes	No
P_7	N	Yes	No	Yes	No	No	No	No	No	No
P_8	H	Yes	Yes	No	Yes	No	Yes	No	Yes	Yes
P_9	H	No	Yes	Yes	No	Yes	Yes	Yes	Yes	No
P_{10}	H	Yes	No	No	Yes	Yes	No	Yes	No	No

In Table 1, abbreviations are used to represent attributes Fever, which is given below:

H: High, N: Normal

The patient P_1 is defined in the COVID-19 table by the following attribute—value set.

(Fever, H), (A dry cough, *Yes)*, (Body aches, No), (Loss of appetite, No), (shortness of breath, Yes), (Fatigue, Yes), (Mucus, No), (Stuffy Nose, Yes), (Nausea, No), (COVID-19, Yes).

The patient P_3 is described as follows. (Fever, H), (A dry cough, *Yes)*, (Body aches, Yes), (Loss of appetite, Yes), (shortness of breath, Yes), (Fatigue, Yes), (Mucus, Yes), (Stuffy Nose, No), (Nausea, Yes), (COVID-19, Yes).

Similarly, patient P_9 is presented as follows.

(Fever, H), (A dry cough, *No)*, (Body aches, Yes), (Loss of appetite, Yes), (shortness of breath, No), (Fatigue, Yes), (Mucus, Yes), (Stuffy Nose, Yes), (Nausea, Yes), (COVID-19, No).

3 Problem Statement

According to Table 1, it is clear that there is need to minimize vagueness in the symptoms of COVID-19 for better predictions and management. Important motivational factor of this study is to optimize the list of potential symptoms responsible for COVID-19. As stated in Table 1, there are 9 symptoms taken into consideration. However, not always all the symptoms contribute to COVID-19 infection. Based on these elementary sets of symptoms patient categorization for COVID-19 can be done effectively with minimal number of symptoms.

4 Design of Proposed Method Based on Rough Sets

In COVID-19 Table 1, patients P_i, for i $\neq$ 5, 7 are indiscernible with respect to the attribute fever and patients P_i, for i $\neq$ 2, 6, 9 are indiscernible for attribute a dry cough. Patients P_1, P_3, P_4, P_8 are indiscernible with respect to the COVID-19. Moreover, patients P_1, P_3, and P_8 are indiscernible with respect to attributes fever, a dry cough and shortness of breath. Patient P_8 has COVID-19, while patient P_5 does not, and they are indiscernible with respect to Fatigue, Mucus, Stuffy Nose, and Nausea. Hence, the COVID-19 cannot be characterized in terms of the attributes like Fatigue, Mucus, Stuffy Nose, and Nausea. Patients P_1 and P_{10} are indiscernible with respect to Fever, a dry cough, body aches, Loss of Appetite, Shortness of Breath, Fatigue, Mucus, Stuffy Nose, and Nausea. Moreover, P_1 and P_{10} are indiscernible with respect to all condition attributes however decision results of COVID-19 infections are different. Therefore, P_1 and P_{10} are the boundary line cases of COVID-19, which cannot be categorized in view of the available information. Now, patients P_1 and P_3 have COVID

-19, but P_1 has no loss of appetite and P_3 has a loss of appetite. Hence, the loss of appetite is not only the characteristics of COVID-19.

By information given in the table, COVID-19 patient is occasionally suffering from body aches. Patients P_3, P_4 and P8 are admitting COVID-19 and they are indiscernible with respect to Fever and dry cough.

Each symptom has different results, so accumulate like symptoms in one set. Such sets are known as elementary sets. Every member of elementary set has same characteristics. These elementary sets form equivalence classes of the data. Therefore, patients having similar characteristics are in one elementary set which helps us for greater understanding. Patients P_3, P_4 and P_8 admit symptoms that facilitate us to classifying them with assurance as having COVID-19. Hence based on symptoms/attributes patients need to classify into elementary sets.

Consider Table 2, which gives the attributes and the corresponding elementary sets. An attribute fever creates two elementary sets {P1, P2, P3, P4, P6, P8, P9, P10}, and {P5, P7}.

Consistent with the research problem, we need to find optimum symptoms that surely decide whether the patient will suffer from COVID-19 or not. Moreover, it is essential to cognize the higher side of symptoms also. According to the rough set theory perspective, it is represented by the lower approximation, upper approximation, accuracy of approximation and class of rough sets. The class of rough sets helps to decide the predictions about whether the patient having COVID-19 or not.

Accordingly, the lower approximation of the set of patients admitting COVID-19, is R_* (X) $\{P_3, P_4, P_8\}$ and R^* (X) $\{P_1, P_2, P_3, P_4, P_5, P_6, P_7, P_8, P_9, P_{10}\}$. Moreover, boundary line cases are P_1 and P_{10}. Consider Table 3, which defines lower approximation, upper approximation, class of rough sets and accuracy of approximation for different sets B.

Table 2 Attributes and corresponding elementary sets

Sr. No.	Attributes	Elementary sets
1	Fever	$\{P_1, P_2, P_3, P_4, P_6, P_8, P_9, P_{10}\}$, $\{P_5, P_7\}$
2	A Dry Cough	$\{P_1, P_3, P_4, P_5, P_7, P_8, P_{10}\}$, $\{P_2, P_6, P_9\}$
3	Body Aches	$\{P_2, P_3, P_4, P_5, P_6, P_8, P_9\}$, $\{P_1, P_7, P_{10}\}$
4	Loss of Appetite	$\{P_2, P_3, P_5, P_7, P_9\}$ $\{P_1, P_4, P_6, P_8, P_{10}\}$
5	Shortness of Breath	$\{P_1, P_2, P_3, P_8, P_{10}\}$. $\{P_4, P_5, P_6, P_7, P_9\}$
6	Fatigue	$\{P_1, P_3, P_4, P_6, P_9, P_{10}\}$, $\{P_2, P_5, P_7, P_8\}$
7	Mucus	$\{P_2, P_3, P_5, P_8, P_9\}$, $\{P_1, P_4, P_6, P_7, P_{10}\}$
8	Stuffy Nose	$\{P_2, P_3, P_5, P_7, P_8\}$, $\{P_1, P_4, P_6, P_9, P_{10}\}$
9	Nausea	$\{P_2, P_3, P_5, P_6, P_8, P_9\}$, $\{P_1, P_4, P_7, P_{10}\}$
10	COVID-19	$\{P_3, P_4, P_8\}$, $\{P_1, P_2, P_5, P_6, P_7, P_9, P_{10}\}$
11	Fever and dry cough	$\{P_1, P_3, P_4, P_8, P_{10}\}$, $\{P_2, P_6, P_9\}$, $\{P_5, P_7\}$
12	Dry Cough and Shortness of breath	$\{P_1, P_3, P_8, P_{10}\}$, $\{P_2\}$, $\{P_4, P_5, P_7\}$, $\{P_6, P_9\}$,

Table 3 Class and accuracy of approximations

Sr. No.	Set B	Lower approximation	Upper approximation	Class of rough sets	Accuracy of approximation
1	Fever	Φ	$U-\{P_5, P_7\} \neq U$	Internally B-indefinable	0
2	A Dry Cough	Φ	$\{P_1, P_3, P_4, P_5, P_7, P_8, P_{10}\}, \neq U$	Internally B-indefinable	0
3	Body Aches	Φ	U	Totally B-indefinable	0
4	Loss of Appetite	Φ	U	Totally B-indefinable	0
5	Shortness of Breath	Φ	U	Totally B-indefinable	0
6	Fatigue	Φ	U	Totally B-indefinable	0
7	Mucus	Φ	U	Totally B-indefinable	0
8	Stuffy Nose	Φ	U	Totally B-indefinable	0
9	Nausea	Φ	U	Totally B-indefinable	0
10	COVID 19	$\{P_3, P_4, P_8\}$	$\{P_1, P_3, P_4, P_8\}$	Roughly B-definable	3/4
11	Fever and dry cough	Φ	$\{P_1, P_3, P_4, P_7, P_8, P_{10}\}$	Internally B-indefinable	0
12	Dry Cough and Shortness of breath	Φ	$\{P_1, P_3, P_4, P_5, P_7\ P_8, P_{10}\}$,	Internally B-indefinable	0

From Table 3, for COVID-19 the class of rough set is roughly B-definable. Therefore, it means that we are able to decide, whether they belong to X or −X, for some elements of U, using B.

For Fever and dry cough as well as Dry Cough and Shortness of breath, the class of rough set is internally B-indefinable. Hence, we are competent to approve whether some elements of the set U have its place to −X, but we are not able to conclude whether it belongs to X or not, using attributes in B The rough class is totally B-indefinable for attributes Body aches, Loss of appetite, shortness of breath, Fatigue, Mucus, Stuffy nose and Nausea. Consequently, it is impotent to approve for any element of the set U, whether it belongs to X or -X by using B.

For all attributes $\alpha_B\ (X)\ <\ 1$, So X is the rough (vague) set with respect to B

A. *Decision Tables and Decision Algorithms*

The information table is classified into two classes of attributes, known as condition and decision attributes.

From Table 1, attributes fever, A dry cough, Body aches, Loss of appetite,, shortness of breath, Fatigue, Mucus, Stuffy nose, Nausea are called condition attributes, while COVID-19 as the decision attributes. Each row of the COVID-19 table governs a decision rule,

A decision rule is determined by each row of COVID-19 table, which states decisions or actions that would be taken when the conditions of the corresponding attributes are satisfied. From Table 1, the condition (Fever, H), (A dry cough, Yes), (Body aches, Yes), (Loss of appetite, Yes), (shortness of breath, Yes), (Fatigue, Yes), (Mucus, Yes), (Stuffy Nose, No), (Nausea, Yes), concludes uniquely the decision (COVID-19, Yes).

In a decision table, objects are used as labels of decision rules. Decision rules 1 and 10 have the same conditions in the decision table, but they have different decisions. A label of decision table in which decisions are different but decision rules are equal is called the inconsistent of conflicting or nondeterministic. If equal decision rules give the same decisions, then it is called consistent or deterministic. The consistent decisions are also known as the sure rules and the inconsistent decisions are called non-sure rules.

In a decision table, the number of consistent rules to all rules is called the consistency factor of the decision table. The consistency factor is denoted by γ (R, D), where R is the conditions and D is the decision attributes. Therefore, if γ (R, D) = 1, then the decision table is called consistent, otherwise inconsistent. For COVID-19 Table 1, γ (R, D) = 10/10 = 1, hence the decision table of COVID-19 is consistent. The decision rules are logical statements. It is presented as "If ... then ... rules". For example, if (Fever, H), (A dry cough, Yes), (Body aches, Yes), (Loss of appetite, Yes), (shortness of breath, Yes), (Fatigue, Yes), (Mucus, Yes), (Stuffy Nose, No), (Nausea, Yes), then (COVID-19, Yes).

A decision algorithm is the set of decision rules. The decision algorithm is nothing but a set of implications (logical expressions).

5 Results and Discussions

From COVID-19 Table 1, it is perceived that, for a few observations,

If (Fatigue, No), (Mucus, Yes), (Stuffy Nose, No), (Nausea, Yes), then (COVID-19, No) for patient P2. And for patient P8, If (Fatigue, No), (Mucus, Yes), (Stuffy Nose, No), (Nausea, Yes), then (COVID-19, Yes). That is for patients P2 and P8, the above conditions are the same but decisions are different and these patients are not on the boundary. Moreover, if (Fatigue, No), (Mucus, No), (Stuffy Nose, No), (Nausea, No), then (COVID-19, No) and if (Fatigue, Yes), (Mucus, Yes), (Stuffy Nose, Yes), (Nausea, Yes), then (COVID-19, No).

Therefore, the above four attributes will not decide, whether the patient is having COVID-19 or not. Thus, the above four attributes can be removed from the set of attributes. Similarly, we can remove body pains and loss of appetite from the table. Thus, the new reduced Table 4 will be as follows

Table 4 Reduced COVID-19 symptoms analysis

Patients	Fever	A dry Cough	Shortness of Breath	COVID-19
P_1	H	Yes	Yes	Yes
P_2	H	No	Yes	No
P_3	H	Yes	Yes	Yes
P_4	H	Yes	No	Yes
P_5	N	Yes	No	No
P_6	H	No	No	No
P_7	N	Yes	No	No
P_8	H	Yes	Yes	Yes
P_9	H	No	No	No
P_{10}	H	Yes	Yes	No

As a result, it is concluded from Table 4 as follows.

1. If the patient has Fever, a dry cough and shortness of breath then out of four such patients, three patients have COVID-19 and one patient has not. The probability of the patient having Fever, a dry cough and shortness of breath with symptoms COVID-19, is ¾ = 0.75.
2. If the patient has a normal fever, then the patient has no any chance of COVID-19, the probability of having COVID-19 is 0.
3. If the patient is suffering from a dry cough then the probability of having COVID-19 is 4/7 = 0.57.
4. If we remove boundary cases and if the patient is having Fever, a dry cough and shortness of breath, then the corresponding probability is 1.
5. If any two attributes out of three are absent in Table 4, then the patient has no COVID-19.
6. If the patient is having any two attributes, then the probability of having COVID-19 is 2/3 = 0.67.

The above six observations help us to calculate the probability of having COVID-19. An application of rough set theory has optimized the number of symptoms responsible for COVID-19 and in the sequel it will also contribute to better and effective decision making. The application of rough sets theory also helps to investigate whether particular symptoms belong to the decision set or not and also the accuracy of observations is calculated and analyzed.

6 Conclusion

In many cases, it seems that there are so many characteristics of the activity but the decision depends upon only a few of them. We have initiated the set of symptoms of the worldwide pandemic COVID-19. The decision table assisted to decide whether the particular patient admits COVID-19 or not by observing common characteristics. The rough set facets facilitated to remove non-important attributes and recognize the foremost attributes which predict resilient decision. Moreover, the probability of having COVID-19 is offered by considering different circumstances. The objective of this work is conquered by reducing the number of symptoms of COVID-19. This symptoms-based prediction could help us for better decision making and management.

Conflict of interest: On behalf of all authors, the corresponding author states that there is no conflict of interest.

References

1. WHO. Coronavirus disease (COVID-2019) situation reports-129. 2020 [cited 2020 May]; Available from https://www.who.int/docs/default-source/coronaviruse/situation-reports/20200528-covid-19-sitrep-129.pdf?sfvrsn=5b154880_2
2. Mahalle, Parikshit N, Nilesh P Sable, Mahalle NP, Shinde GR (2020) Predictive Analytics of COVID-19 using information, communication and technologies
3. Mahalle P, Kalamkar AB, Dey N, Chaki J, Shinde GR (2020) Forecasting models for Coronavirus (COVID-19): A Survey of the State-of-the-Art. (2020) SN COMPUT. SCI. 1, 197 (2020). https://doi.org/10.1007/s42979-020-00209-9
4. Shinde, Rahul G, Kalamkar AB, Mahalle PN, Dey N (2020) Data analytics for coronavirus disease (COVID-19) outbreak. Publisher: CRC Press, ISBN: 9780367558468
5. Dey N, Rajinikant V, Fong SJ, Kaiser MS, Mahmud M (2020) Social-group-optimization assisted Kapur's entropy and morphological segmentation for automated detection of COVID-19 infection from computed tomography images
6. Sameni R (2020) Mathematical modeling of epidemic diseases; a case study of the COVID-19 coronavirus. arXiv preprint arXiv:2003.11371
7. Fong SJ, Li G, Dey N, Crespo RG, Herrera-Viedma E (2020) Composite Monte Carlo decision making under high uncertainty of novel coronavirus epidemic using hybridized deep learning and fuzzy rule induction. Appl Soft Comput, 106282
8. Santosh KC (2020) AI-driven tools for coronavirus outbreak: need of active learning and cross-population train/test models on multitudinal/multimodal data. J Med Syst 44(5):1–5
9. Roda WC, Varughese MB, Han D, Li MY (2020) Why is it difficult to accurately predict the COVID-19 epidemic? Infectious Disease Model
10. Huang R, Liu M, Ding Y (2020) Spatial-temporal distribution of COVID-19 in China and its prediction: a data-driven modeling analysis. J Infect Dev Countries 14(3):246–253
11. Bhattacharjee S (2020) Statistical investigation of relationship between spread of coronavirus disease (COVID-19) and environmental factors based on study of four mostly affected places of China and five mostly affected places of Italy. arXiv preprint arXiv:2003.11277
12. Dowd JB, Andriano L, Brazel DM, Rotondi V, Block P, Ding X, Liu Y, Mills MC (2020) Demographic science aids in understanding the spread and fatality rates of COVID-19. Proceedings of the National Academy of Sciences 117, no. 18, pp 9696–9698
13. Acharjya D, Anitha A (2017) A comparative study of statistical and rough computing models in predictive data analysis. Int J Ambient Comput Intell (IJACI) 8(2):32–51
14. Acharjya DP (2020) Behavioural intention of customers towards smartwatches in an ambient environment using soft computing: an integrated SEM-PLS and fuzzy rough set approach. Int J Ambient Comput Intell (IJACI) 11(2):80–111
15. Roy P, Goswami S, Chakraborty S, Azar AT, Dey N (2014) Image segmentation using rough set theory: a review. Int J Rough Sets Data Analys (IJRSDA) 1(2):62–74

16. Ripon SH, Kamal S, Hossain S, Dey N (2016) Theoretical analysis of different classifiers under reduction rough data set: a brief proposal. Int J Rough Sets Data Analys (IJRSDA) 3(3):1–20
17. Chowdhuri S, Roy P, Goswami S, Azar AT, Dey N (2014) Rough set based ad hoc network: a review. Int J Serv Sci Manag Eng Technol (IJSSMET) 5(4):66–76
18. Li Z, Shi K, Dey N, Ashour AS, Wang D, Balas VE…Shi F (2017). Rule-based back propagation neural networks for various precision rough set presented KANSEI knowledge prediction: a case study on shoe product form features extraction. Neural Comput Appl 28(3):613–630
19. Mardani A, Nilashi M, Antucheviciene J, Tavana M, Bausys R, Ibrahim O (2020) Recent fuzzy generalisations of rough sets theory: a systematic review and methodological critique of the literature. Complexity 2017
20. Maeda Y, Senoo K, Tanaka H (1999) Interval density function in conflict analysis. In: Zhong N, Skowron A, Ohsuga S (eds) New directions in rough sets. Springer, Data Mining and Granular-Soft Computing, pp 382–389
21. Symptoms of Coronavirus [cited 2020 May]. https://www.webmd.com/lung/covid-19-symptoms

COVID-19 Detection via Wavelet Entropy and Biogeography-Based Optimization

Xujing Yao and Ji Han

Abstract Since the end of 2019, the COVID-19 virus has swept the world, bringing great impact to various fields and gaining wide attention from all walks of life. COVID-19 is known to have a long incubation period. Thus, in terms of virus detection, it's very time consuming and labor-intensive. Artificial intelligence can analyze CT scan images and assist in detection of patients, which is of great help to realize rapid, effective and safe detection of COVID-19. In this research, a dataset of 132 samples was collected from the Fourth People's Hospital of Huai'an City. One part of 66 patients with novel coronavirus pneumonia and the other part of 66 healthy people. This experiment uses Wavelet Entropy as a feature extraction method, K-fold as a validation method that reports unbiased performances, Biogeography-based Optimization as a training algorithm and Single-hidden-layer as a classifier. The proposed model achieves good performance with mean sensitivity of 72.97 ± 2.96%, specificity of 74.93 ± 2.39%, precision of 74.48 ± 1.34%, accuracy of 73.95 ± 0.98%, F1 score of 73.65 ± 1.33% and Matthews correlation coefficient of 47.99 ± 2.00%. The results confirmed that this artificial intelligence model can well complete the detection task of COVID-19 via Wavelet Entropy and Biogeography-based Optimization.

Keywords COVID-19 · Chest CT · Wavelet entropy · Biogeography-based optimization · K-fold Cross-Validation · Single-hidden-layer

---

X. Yao (✉) · J. Han
School of Informatics, University of Leicester, Leicester LE1 7RH, UK
e-mail: xy147@leicester.ac.uk

X. Yao
Department of Medical Imaging, The Fourth People's Hospital of Huai'an, Huai'an, Jiangsu 223002, China

J. Han
School of Computer Science and Technology, Henan Polytechnic University, Jiaozuo, Henan 454000, People's Republic of China

K. C. Santosh and A. Joshi (eds.), *COVID-19: Prediction, Decision-Making, and its Impacts*, Lecture Notes on Data Engineering and Communications Technologies 60, https://doi.org/10.1007/978-981-15-9682-7_8

1 Introduction

COVID-19 is an acute infectious pneumonia caused by a novel coronavirus that has never been found in humans before. The virus shares a structural similarity of 87.1% [1] to the SARS-related virus found in bats, and 79.5% [2] to the SARS virus. Novel coronavirus is parallel to SARS coronavirus, which means, they belong to the same family of viruses but are not the same.

On 30 January 2020, the world health organization (WHO) declared the COVID-19 outbreak a public health emergency (PHEIC) of international concern. Based on the current epidemiological investigation, the incubation period is from 1 day to 14 days, in most cases from 3 days to 7 days [3]. The patient in the incubation period has no difference in appearance when compared to normal people but is contagious. The initial symptoms of the patients are fever, dry cough, fatigue, and will gradually appear breathing difficulties and other serious manifestations. Asymptomatic infected persons can also be a source of infection [4–9].

Novel coronavirus specific reverse transcription-polymerase chain reaction (RT-PCR) is the most common standard method for novel coronavirus detection. However, its tests can take up to two days to complete and may require repeated tests to rule out potential false negatives [10]. In order to improve the speed and accuracy of detecting novel coronavirus, the medical community believes that chest computed tomography (CT) scan can be utilized as a useful tool for early diagnosis of novel coronavirus suspected infection. Chest CT is a common and basic diagnostic technique for pneumonia. This technique uses X-ray CT to examine the chest. Fang et al. [10] and his team members made a comparison between the sensitivity of Chest CT and RT-PCR for detecting COVID-19. The results reveal that utilizing Chest CT to screen the COVID-19 patient is an effective way, especially when the patient is tested negative in RT-PCR.

The research of Yildiz et al. [11] presented a feature extraction method in combination of discrete wavelet transform (DWT) and entropy. They first utilized DWT to separate those achieved EEG signals to sub-bands and then applied Shannon entropy algorithm to calculate each subband's entropy.

Simon [12] with his team put forward a concept of Biogeography-based Optimization (BBO), which is inspired by the principle of biogeography. It can be understood that through the migration and drift of species between geographical areas, nature can finally reach a balanced state. The species here can actually be viewed as information, which is essentially the dependent variable.

This paper intends to propose a method on the basis of wavelet entropy and BBO. The classification process can be very complex when dealing with a large number of high-dimensional feature vectors due to the reason that some features with redundancy will reduce the classification rate. In addition, reducing the number of features helps the classifier learn more robust solutions and obtain better generalization performance. Thus, our paper prefers utilizing wavelet entropy to efficiently reduce the feature dimension. We also focus on the advantages of BBO algorithm in (i) its own mining ability; (ii) it adopts integer coding; (iii) it takes less time; (iv) it converges quickly; (v) it is not easy to fall into the local optimal.

2 Dataset

The collected dataset can be divided into two parts. One part from COVID-19 patients and the other part from healthy people. The example images are displayed in Fig. 1. The first part is from 66 patients with COVID-19 who were admitted to the Fourth People's Hospital of Huai'an City from January 2020 to March 2020. These patients have both positive nucleic acid test result and complete Chest CT image data. At the same time period, through utilizing systematic random sampling, the second part of another 66 cases was selected from 159 physical examination personnel who have negative nucleic acid test result.

In the observation group, there were 39 male and 27 female COVID-19 patients, aged from 24 to 91 years old, with an average age of 48.00 ± 15.32 years. In the control group, there were 38 males and 28 females from people who passed the normal health checkup, aged from 25 to 72 years, with an average age of 38.44 ± 10.58 years.

For the sake of observation, images are all uploaded onto the medical image Picture Archiving and Communication Systems (PASC). Two professional chest radiologists collectively read the X-ray. They first recorded the distribution, size and shape of the CT appearance of the lesion, and then selected 1-4 CT images from each person. When two professional radiologists differed in their analysis, a senior physician would be consulted to reach an agreement.

The agreed slice level selection method is: for patients with COVID-19, the slice with the largest size and number of lesions was selected; and for normal cases, any level of the slice can be chosen.

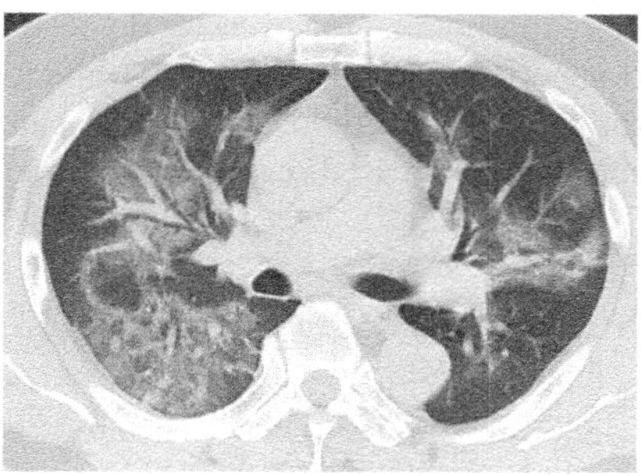
(a) COVID-19 patient

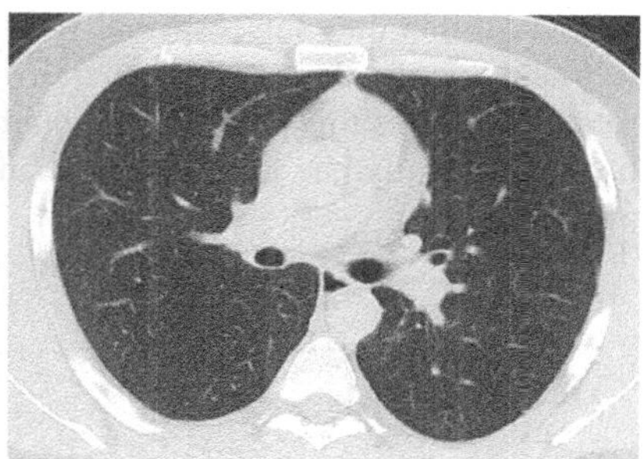
(b) Healthy people

Fig. 1 Illustration of our COVID-19 dataset

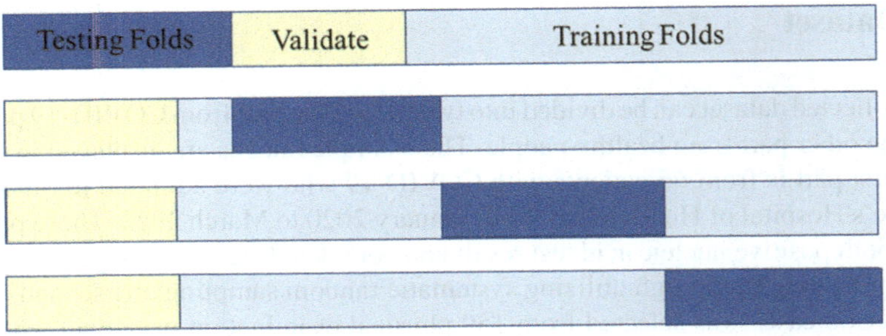

Fig. 2 An illustration of 4-fold cross-validation

2.1 K-Fold Cross-Validation

For the purpose of avoiding the problem of overfitting, K-fold cross-validation technique is developed and applied in many cases [13–18]. In a certain sense, the original dataset was grouped, with one part as training set, one part as validation set and one part as testing set. K-fold cross-validation will randomly divide the training data into k parts and do k times of training. The validation set was set to test the generalization error of the model [19]. An illustration of 4-fold cross-validation is shown in Fig. 2.

Another reason for adopting k-fold in this experiment is that this method is very suitable for processing data sets with only a small amount of data. Without utilizing K-fold cross-validation, testing set will not participate in the training, which wastes this part of data and to some degree fails to optimize the model due to the reason that data determines the upper limit of program performance. Thus, it is significant to make good use of data sets, especially for this experiment. However, we do need the testing set to verify the network generalization performance. K-fold cross-validation successfully solves this problem. Through utilizing this method, all data sets can be utilized, and finally, the model performance can be expressed reasonably by means of averaging [20].

3 Methodology

3.1 Wavelet Entropy

Wavelet transform is a transform analysis method that inherits and develops the idea of Fourier transform (FFT). It effectively solves the previous defect of the inability of the FFT to handle unstable signals. The wavelet transform simply changes the basis of the Fourier transform. It replaces an infinitely long trig basis with a decaying wavelet basis of a finite length. In this way, the frequency can be captured, and the time can be accurately located [21]. The equation of FFT is illustrated in Eq. (1).

The equation for wavelet transform is illustrated in Eq. (2).

$$F(w) = \int_{-\infty}^{\infty} f(t) * e^{-iwt} dt \tag{1}$$

$$WT(s, \tau) = \frac{1}{\sqrt{s}} \int_{-\infty}^{\infty} f(t) * \psi\left(\frac{t - \tau}{s}\right) dt \tag{2}$$

where w refers to frequency, s refers to scale, τ refers to translation.

Wavelet transform can effectively decompose images of different pixels and retain image information [22–27]. However, loads of image features are left after the decomposing, which brings many drawbacks. The first is too many features require lots of storage space. Apart from that, the calculation time takes longer. Thus, the concept of entropy has to be introduced to reduce the dimension of the feature [28]

Entropy is the measurement of the uniformity of a distribution: the higher the entropy, the more uniform the distribution. In information theory, information entropy can explain the degree of chaos of a message, in other words, to determine the amount of information contained in a random data source [29].

Suppose a random variable X, the value of X in dataset D is $X = \{x_1, x_2, \ldots, x_n\}$, $P(R)$ is the probability function, then the entropy is:

$$H(X) = E[I(X)] = E[-\ln(k(X))] \tag{3}$$

where E refers to the expected value.

If D is an infinite set, then the entropy of the random variable X is:

$$H(X) = -\Sigma_i P(X_i) \log_b P(X_i) \tag{4}$$

3.2 *Biogeography-Based Optimization*

The mechanism of biogeographic optimization algorithm updating data mainly depends on two operations: migration and mutation.

There are many physical models for species migration, such as linear model, cosine model, quadratic model and exponential model [30]. As can be seen from Fig. 3, there is a certain relationship between the number of living things in a certain place and the rate of moving in and out. From a theoretical point of view, the in-and-out operation is to update the array according to a particular physical model [31–35].

In order to increase the diversity of the newly generated array, mutation operation is introduced. Mutation operation is similar to genetic algorithm, and the formula is:

Fig. 3 A typical linear migration model

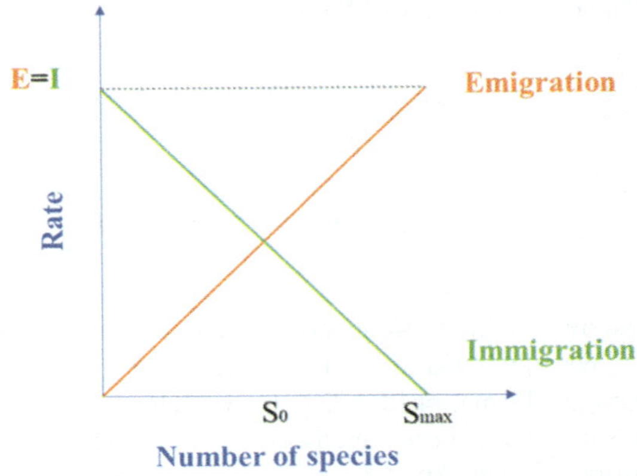

$$m(S) = m_{\max}\left(\frac{1 - P_s}{P_{\max}}\right) \quad (5)$$

where $m_{\max}$ is a predefined mutation-related parameter, representing the maximum mutation rate. $P_{\max}$ is the maximum value of $P(\infty)$ [36].

4 Experiments, Results and Discussion

This experiment uses Wavelet Entropy as feature extraction method, K-fold as validation method which reports unbiased performances, Biogeography-based Optimization as training algorithm and Single-hidden-layer neural network [37, 38] as classifier. The result of our artificial intelligence model is displayed in Table 1.

Our model achieves good performance with mean sensitivity of $72.97 \pm 2.96\%$, specificity of $74.93 \pm 2.39\%$, precision of $74.48 \pm 1.34\%$, accuracy of $73.95 \pm 0.98\%$, F1 score of $73.66 \pm 1.33\%$ and Matthews correlation coefficient of $47.99 \pm 2.00\%$. It is worth mentioning that the accuracy and specificity of our model is much higher than Ai, Yang [39] reported. His team worked on a dataset of Chest CT either, and achieved 65% accuracy and 27% specificity for people aged under 60. This indicates our model provides an efficient and promising way to detect COVID-19.

5 Conclusion

Chest CT is known to be a rapid, non-invasive method. Our artificial intelligence model using Wavelet Entropy and Biogeography-based Optimization is also an efficient method to accomplish the classification task. To conclude, combine these two techniques can help to realize rapid, effective and safe detection of COVID-19, which is of great significance to clinical medicine and society.

Table 1 10 runs of 4-fold cross-validation on our model (Unit: %)

Run	Sen	Spc	Prc	Acc	F1	MCC
1	72.97	72.97	72.96	72.97	72.96	45.95
2	72.30	72.30	72.30	72.30	72.28	44.62
3	72.97	76.35	75.53	74.66	74.20	49.38
4	74.32	74.32	74.32	74.32	74.32	48.65
5	68.92	76.35	74.40	72.64	71.54	45.40
6	70.95	77.70	76.06	74.32	73.40	48.77
7	69.59	78.38	76.33	73.99	72.79	48.17
8	72.30	77.03	75.87	74.66	74.04	49.38
9	75.68	72.30	73.24	73.99	74.41	48.04
10	79.73	71.62	73.74	75.68	76.60	51.56
Mean + SD	72.97 ± 2.96	74.93 ± 2.39	74.48 ± 1.34	73.95 ± 0.98	73.66 ± 1.33	47.99 ± 2.00

(Sen = Sensitivity; Spc = Specificity; Prc = Precision; Acc = Accuracy; F1 = F1 Score; MCC = Matthews correlation coefficient; SD = standard deviation)

References

1. Zhao W et al (2020) Relation between chest CT findings and clinical conditions of coronavirus disease (COVID-19) pneumonia: a multicenter study. Am J Roentgenol 214(5):1072–1077
2. Zheng M et al (2020) Functional exhaustion of antiviral lymphocytes in COVID-19 patients. Cellular Molecu Immunol, 1–3
3. Wen X, Li Y (2020) Anesthesia procedure of emergency operation for patients with suspected or confirmed COVID-19. Surgical Infections 21(3):299
4. Kooraki S et al (2020) Coronavirus (COVID-19) outbreak: what the department of radiology should know. J Amer Colle Radiol
5. Mukherjee H et al (2020) shallow convolutional neural network for COVID-19 outbreak screening using chest X-rays2020
6. Das, D., K. Santosh, and U. Pal, Truncated inception net: COVID-19 outbreak screening using chest X-rays. Physical and engineering sciences in medicine, 2020: p. 1–11
7. Rajinikanth V et al (2020) Harmony-search and otsu based system for coronavirus disease (COVID-19) detection using lung CT scan images. arXiv preprint arXiv:2004.03431
8. Dey N et al (2020) social-group-optimization assisted Kapur's entropy and morphological segmentation for automated detection of COVID-19 infection from computed tomography images
9. Fong SJ, Dey N, Chaki J, Artificial intelligence for coronavirus outbreak
10. Fang Y et al (2020) Sensitivity of chest CT for COVID-19: comparison to RT-PCR. Radiology, 200432
11. Yildiz A et al (2009) Application of adaptive neuro-fuzzy inference system for vigilance level estimation by using wavelet-entropy feature extraction. Expert Syst Appl 36(4):7390–7399
12. Simon D (2008) Biogeography-based optimization. IEEE Trans Evol Comput 12(6):702–713
13. Jiang Y (2018) Exploring a smart pathological brain detection method on pseudo Zernike moment. Multimedia Tools Appl 77(17):22589–22604
14. Hou X-X (2018) Voxelwise detection of cerebral microbleed in CADASIL patients by leaky rectified linear unit and early stopping. Multimedia Tools Appl 77(17):21825–21845
15. Cheng H (2018) Multiple sclerosis identification based on fractional Fourier entropy and a modified Jaya algorithm. Entropy 20(4)

16. Zhan T (2016) Pathological brain detection by artificial intelligence in magnetic resonance imaging scanning. Progress Electromagn Res 156:105–133
17. Phillips P (2015) Pathological brain detection in magnetic resonance imaging scanning by wavelet entropy and hybridization of biogeography-based optimization and particle swarm optimization. Progress Electromagn Res 152:41–58
18. Chen X-Q (2016) Fractal dimension estimation for developing pathological brain detection system based on Minkowski-Bouligand method. IEEE Access 4:5937–5947
19. Moore AW (2001) Cross-validation for detecting and preventing overfitting. School of Computer Science Carneigie Mellon University
20. Yadav S, Shukla S (2016) Analysis of k-fold cross-validation over hold-out validation on colossal datasets for quality classification. In: 2016 IEEE 6th International conference on advanced computing (IACC). IEEE
21. Rao R (2002) Wavelet transforms. Encyclopedia of imaging science and technology
22. Qian P (2018) Cat Swarm Optimization applied to alcohol use disorder identification. Multimedia Tools Appl 77(17):22875–22896
23. Li Y-J (2018) Single slice based detection for Alzheimer's disease via wavelet entropy and multilayer perceptron trained by biogeography-based optimization. Multimedia Tools Appl 77(9):10393–10417
24. Gorriz JM (2018) Multivariate approach for Alzheimer's disease detection using stationary wavelet entropy and predator-prey particle swarm optimization. J Alzheimers Dis 65(3):855–869
25. Dong Z (2017) Synthetic minority oversampling technique and fractal dimension for identifying multiple sclerosis. Fractals 25(4)
26. Nayak DR (2017) Detection of unilateral hearing loss by stationary wavelet entropy. CNS & Neurological Disorders-Drug Targets 16(2):15–24
27. Gorriz JM, Ramírez J (2016) Wavelet entropy and directed acyclic graph support vector machine for detection of patients with unilateral hearing loss in MRI scanning. Front Comput Neurosci 10
28. Rosso OA et al (2001) Wavelet entropy: a new tool for analysis of short duration brain electrical signals. J Neurosci Methods 105(1):65–75
29. Gray RM (2011) Entropy and information theory. Springer Science & Business Media
30. Ma H et al (2012) Biogeography-based optimization with ensemble of migration models for global numerical optimization. In: 2012 IEEE congress on evolutionary computer. IEEE
31. Li P, Liu G (2017) Pathological brain detection via wavelet packet tsallis entropy and real-coded biogeography-based optimization. Fundamenta Informat 151(1–4):275–291
32. Wu X (2016) Smart detection on abnormal breasts in digital mammography based on contrast-limited adaptive histogram equalization and chaotic adaptive real-coded biogeography-based optimization. Simulation 92(9):873–885
33. Wu J (2016) Fruit classification by biogeography-based optimization and feedforward neural network. Expert Syst 33(3):239–253
34. Wei L (2015) Fruit classification by wavelet-entropy and feedforward neural network trained by fitness-scaled chaotic ABC and biogeography-based optimization. Entropy 17(8):5711–5728
35. Yang G (2016) Automated classification of brain images using wavelet-energy and biogeography-based optimization. Multimedia Tools Appl 75(23):15601–15617
36. Kumaran J, Ravi G (2015) Long-term sector-wise electrical energy forecasting using artificial neural network and biogeography-based optimization. Electric Power Compon Syst 43(11):1225–1235
37. Feng C (2015) Feed-forward neural network optimized by hybridization of PSO and ABC for abnormal brain detection. Int J Imaging Syst Technol 25(2):153–164
38. Rao RV, Liu A, Wei L (2017) Abnormal Breast Detection in Mammogram Images by Feed-forward neural network trained by jaya algorithm. Fundamenta Informaticae 151(1–4):191–211
39. Ai T et al (2020) Correlation of Chest CT and RT-PCR Testing in Coronavirus Disease 2019 (COVID-19) in China: A Report of 1014 Cases. Radiology, p 200642

Machine Learning in Fighting Pandemics: A COVID-19 Case Study

Mufti Mahmud and M. Shamim Kaiser

Abstract In today's digitised world, machine learning (ML) has been playing a very important role in identifying patterns from the ever-growing amount of data made available by the devices and sensors used in the day-to-day activities. Applications of ML have enriched many fields directly connected to our daily lives including education, finance, governance, healthcare, security and surveillance, etc. Its applications can also be extended in facilitating the management of pandemics, especially when the world is experiencing an unprecedented pandemic caused by the novel coronavirus disease (COVID-19). This chapter aims to provide an account of how ML can be utilised in fighting pandemics in general, with a focus on the COVID-19.

Keywords Novel coronavirus · Pandemic management · Multi-sensor data · Infection management · Disease spread management

1 Introduction

Since December 2019, the world has experienced a new disease, known as COVID-19, caused by the novel coronavirus which has been identified as Severe Acute Respiratory Syndrome Coronavirus 2 (SARS-CoV-2) [1]. This has caused havoc around the world with over 5.5 million people infected and more than 348 K dead as of 25 May 2020 [2]. Due to the severity of spread and infection, this disease has been declared as a global pandemic by the World Health Organization (WHO) on 11 March 2020 [3].

Pandemics are important threats to life and health and require great efforts to be contained and made less serious. The difficulties in their management depend

M. Mahmud (✉)
Department of Computer Science, Nottingham Trent University, Clifton Lane, Nottingham NG11 8NS, UK
e-mail: muftimahmud@gmail.com; mufti.mahmud@ntu.ac.uk

M. S. Kaiser
Institute of Information Technology, Jahangirnagar University, Savar, Dhaka 1342, Bangladesh
e-mail: mskaiser@juniv.edu

K. C. Santosh and A. Joshi (eds.), *COVID-19: Prediction, Decision-Making, and its Impacts*, Lecture Notes on Data Engineering and Communications Technologies 60, https://doi.org/10.1007/978-981-15-9682-7_9

on multiple factors, starting with the unpredictability and mutability that characterizes them, to arrive at the indispensability of international and national coordination, especially in the current situation of globalization and rapid interconnection of people and goods. A further difficulty consists of providing timely, comprehensible and as accurate information as possible both to health workers and to the general population, keeping the level of awareness sufficiently high to be able to detect suspicious or ascertained cases early, without however raising alarms. The refutation of false news not supported by reliable sources is also very important to avoid further personal, social and economic damage: anxiety and in some cases psychosis, the result of uncontrolled and alarmist news, can provoke totally unjustified discrimination of entire groups population, even only for ethnicity and damage important economic sectors (such as tourism, trade and catering) [4]. In addition, the excess of prevention which is not effective can overload and clog health services, induce unnecessary health costs (for example, protective masks, non-indicated diagnostic tests, unnecessary visits), subtracting important resources. On the other hand, all those non-medical individual and social behaviours at minimal or zero cost, which are also useful for preventing and mitigating other pathologies and for strengthening cohesion and social and psychological support, which are also fundamental in a moment of crisis, especially in individualistic societies such as the western ones.

Now, it is clear that these events of the past few weeks have led to an impressive change in the world. The world has never been so helpless in the last century since the Spanish Flu pandemic in 1918 caused by the H1N1 virus [5]. But since then, the field of medical science has witnessed unprecedented improvement in treating diseases and developing cures [6]. Also, other technological innovations have contributed in accelerating healthcare provisions and delivery during the last decades [7]. In this advanced computing, data analytics and artificial intelligence also have played an important role [8–11]. Also, machine learning (ML) has been successfully applied to tasks such as biological data mining [12, 13], image analysis [14], financial forecasting [15], anomaly detection [16], disease detection [17, 18, 19], natural language processing [20] and strategic game playing [21]. Therefore, in this chapter we will explore the application of ML in supporting the COVID-19 pandemic.

2 Vulnerability Assessment

Long before COVID-19 became a public health problem in the form of a pandemic, there have been regular efforts from all public health systems, especially in the developed world, to perform assessment of the social determinants of health; thus identifying population who are at the risk of such public health problem [22]. These efforts allow identification of many social risk factors such as being homeless or living in solitude, therefore without the possibility of contacting family or friends in case of need. This opens possibilities to use advanced data science and ML tools and techniques in detecting the most vulnerable population [23]. Therefore, by crossing social risk data with health risk data, for example, age or conditions such as diabetes and lung disease, the ML-based artificial intelligence (AI) system aims to identify those who are the most vulnerable to COVID-19 infection. Once the high-risk peoples have been identified, specific health service providers who have already established trust relationships with them in the past will be able to contact them to build awareness among them to limit the spread of the virus and provide them with necessary alimentation and related support to stay safe.

3 Patient Screening

The area where the most technological support can be delivered is in the process of identifying the coronavirus disease [24]. There are several multi-national incorporations who have devoted their support in developing ML and AI-based solutions in detecting the disease [25, 26]. An early example has been set by the technology giants, including Alibaba, Apple, Baidu, DiDi, Huawei, Microsoft and Tencent, who have developed or promised development of new diagnostic tools based on AI which are capable of diagnosing new cases of coronavirus [27]. One specific case has been the AI system developed by Alibaba, which has reached an accuracy rate of up to 96% in detecting coronavirus and this has allowed a reduction in the waiting times of the traditional swab based detection tests since it only takes 20 s to obtain the test results [28].

The ML model developed by Alibaba to perform this scan has been trained, according to Alibaba Damo Academy researchers, with a sample of over 5,000 Coronavirus positive cases. The advantages in this case favour not only the population but also the hospitals, which are lightened by an otherwise much longer activity, quickly distinguishing between COVID-19 and pneumonia cases [28].

4 Drug Development

Another potential application area where ML has been practically employed in fighting pandemics is supporting the drug development process. There are several pharmaceutical giants such as Eli Lilly and Incyte have already received approval in rolling-out treatment of rheumatoid arthritis and is being studied for other indications. This has been facilitated by AI companies such as BenevolentAI who have applied ML and AI at every stage of the drug discovery process: from the generation of hypotheses to the initial phase of clinical development [29]. The company announced that baricitinib, identified using ML and AI as a potential treatment for COVID-19, is entering a randomized controlled trial phase with the U.S. National Institute of Allergy and Infectious Diseases [30].

5 Conclusions

AI and ML can be proven to be a fundamental tool to identify and protect the most vulnerable people. A strategy that can also be taken as an example by other health systems: if, in fact, there are patient data available relating to their social conditions, in addition to the clinical ones, ML approaches could identify patients at risk in emergency situations like this. Even if only medical information were available, thanks to AI algorithms, the data could be used to identify those who, on the basis of medical parameters, present a greater risk. And this would mean contributing to safeguarding everyone else's health. Especially during an epidemic. Also, it can contribute in detecting the disease itself and facilitate the development of a cure such as vaccine and drugs.

References

1. Atkinson B, Petersen E (2020) SARS-CoV-2 shedding and infectivity. Lancet 395(10233):1339–1340
2. Worldometer (2020) Coronavirus updates. https://www.worldometers.info/coronavirus/ Accessed 25 May 2020
3. World Health Organisation (2020) WHO director-general's opening remarks at the media briefing on COVID-19 11 March 2020. https://www.who.int/dg/speeches/detail/who-director-general-s-opening-remarks-at-the-media-briefing-on-covid-19---11-march-2020 Accessed 25 May 2020
4. Satu MS, Khan MI, Mahmud M, Uddin S, Summers MA, Quinn JM, Moni MA (2020) TClustVID: a novel machine learning classification model to investigate topics and sentiment in COVID-19 Tweets. medRxiv. 2020:1–31. https://doi.org/10.1101/2020.08.04.20167973
5. CDC (2020) 1918 pandemic (H1N1 Virus). https://www.cdc.gov/flu/pandemic-resources/1918-pandemic-h1n1.html. Accessed 25 May 2020
6. Thomson WAR, Richardson RG, et al. (2020) History of medicine. Encyclopædia Britannica. https://www.britannica.com/science/history-of-medicine Accessed on 25 May 2020
7. Timmermann C, Anderson J (2006) Devices, designs and the history of technology in medicine. In: Timmermann C, Anderson J (eds) Devices and Designs: Medical Technologies in Historical Perspective. Palgrave Macmillan UK, London, pp 1–14
8. Clancey WJ, Shortliffe EH (1984) Readings in medical artificial intelligence: the first decade. Addison-Wesley Longman Publishing Co. Inc, Boston, MA
9. Santosh KC (2020) AI-driven tools for coronavirus outbreak: need of active learning and cross-population train/test models on multitudinal/multimodal data. J Med Syst 44:93
10. Fong SJ, Dey N, Chaki J (2020) Artificial Intelligence for Coronavirus Outbreak. Springer, Singapore
11. Fong SJ, Dey N, Chaki J (2020) AI-enabled technologies that fight the coronavirus outbreak. In: Artificial intelligence for coronavirus outbreak. Springer, Singapore, , pp 23–45
12. Mahmud M, Kaiser MS, Hussain A, Vassanelli S (2018) Applications of deep learning and reinforcement learning to biological data. IEEE Trans Neural Netw Learn Syst 29(6):2063–2079
13. Mahmud M, Kaiser MS, McGinnity TM, Hussain A (2020) Deep learning in mining biological data. Cogn Comput 1–36, doi: 10.1007/s12559-020-09773-x
14. Ali HM, Kaiser MS, Mahmud M (2019) Application of convolutional neural network in segmenting brain regions from MRI data. In: International conference on brain information. Springer, pp136–146

15. Orojo O, Tepper J, McGinnity TM, Mahmud M (2019) A multi-recurrent network for crude oil price prediction. In: Proceedings of 2019 IEEE symposium series on computational intelligence (SSCI), pp 2953–2958
16. Yahaya SW, Lotfi A, Mahmud M (2019) A consensus novelty detection ensemble approach for anomaly detection in activities of daily living. Appl Soft Comput 83:105613
17. Noor MBT, Zenia NZ, Kaiser MS, Mahmud M, Mamun SA (2019) Detecting neurodegenerative disease from mri: a brief review on a deep learning perspective. In: International conference on brain information. Springer, pp 115–125
18. Miah Y, Prima CNE, Seema SJ, Mahmud M, Kaiser MS (2020) Performance comparison of machine learning techniques in identifying dementia from open access clinical datasets. In: Proceedings of ICACIN 2020. Springer, Singapore, pp 79–89
19. Noor MBT, Zenia NZ, Kaiser MS, Mamun SA, Mahmud M (2020) Application of deep learning in detecting neurological disorders from magnetic resonance images: a survey on the detection of Alzheimer's disease, Parkinson's disease and schizophrenia. Brain Inf 7:11
20. Rabby G, Azad S, Mahmud M, Zamli KZ, Rahman MM (2020) Teket: a tree-based unsupervised keyphrase extraction technique. Cogn Comput 12(4):811-833
21. Silver D et al (2016) (2016) Mastering the game of go with deep neural networks and tree search. Nature 529(7587):484
22. Jesmin S, Kaiser MS, Mahmud M (2020) Artificial and internet of healthcare things based alzheimer care during COVID 19. In: International Conference on Brain Informatics. Springer, pp 263–274
23. Uddin MS, Nasseef MT, Mahmud M, AlArjani A (2020) Mathematical modelling in prediction of novel coronavirus (COVID-19). Trans Dyn. Preprints 2020:2020090757. https://doi.org/10.20944/preprints202009.0757.v1
24. Arifeen MM, Al Mamun A, Kaiser MS, Mahmud M (2020) Blockchain-enable contact tracing for preserving user privacy during COVID-19 outbreak. Preprints 2020:2020070502. https://doi.org/10.20944/preprints202007.0502.v1
25. Dey N, Rajinikanth V, Fong SJ, Kaiser MS, Mahmud M (2020) Social group optimization–assisted Kapur's entropy and morphological segmentation for automated detection of COVID-19 infection from computed tomography images. Cogn Comput 12(5):1011–1023
26. Aradhya VNM, Mahmud M, Agarwal B, Guru DS, Kaiser MS (2021) One shot cluster based approach for the detection of COVID-19 from chest X-ray images. Cogn Comput 1–8 [epub ahead of print]
27. Kharpal A. (2020) China's giants from Alibaba to Tencent ramp up health tech efforts to battle coronavirus. https://www.cnbc.com/2020/03/04/coronavirus-china-alibaba-tencent-baidu-boost-health-tech-efforts.html Accessed 25 May 2020.
28. Henan S (2020) Alibaba says AI can identify coronavirus infections with 96% accuracy. https://asia.nikkei.com/Spotlight/Coronavirus/Alibaba-says-AI-can-identify-coronavirus-infections-with-96-accuracy. Accessed 25 May 2020
29. Stebbing J et al (2020) COVID-19: combining antiviral and anti-inflammatory treatments. Lancet Infect Dis 20:400–402
30. Richardson P et al (2020) Baricitinib as potential treatment for 2019-nCoV acute respiratory disease. Lancet 395:e30–e31

Healthcare Robots to Combat COVID-19

M. Shamim Kaiser, Shamim Al Mamun, Mufti Mahmud, and Marzia Hoque Tania

Abstract Advancement in robotic technology triggered its usability in the next generation healthcare system. Healthcare robots are expected to assist clinicians and healthcare professionals at all settings by monitoring patient's physiological conditions in real time, facilitating advanced intervention such as robotic surgery, supporting patient care at the hospital and home, dispensing medication, assisting patients with cognition challenges and disabilities, keeping company to geriatric and physically/mentally challenged patients and hospital building management such as disinfecting places. Thus, the robotic agent can enhance healthcare experiences by reducing patient care work and strenuous/repetitive manual tasks. The robotic applications can also be elongated in supporting the healthcare system for the management of pandemics like novel coronavirus (COVID-19) infection and upcoming pandemics. Such applications include collecting the sample from a patient for screening, disinfecting the hospital, supply logistics, and food to the infected patient, collect physiological conditions. This chapter aims to provide an overview of various types of assistive robots employed for healthcare services especially in fighting pandemic and natural disasters.

Keywords Physically and mentally challenged · IoT · Patient care · Pandemics

M. S. Kaiser (✉) · S. Al Mamun
Institute of Information Technology, Jahangirnagar University, Savar, Dhaka 1342, Bangladesh
e-mail: mskaiser@juniv.edu

S. Al Mamun
e-mail: shamim@juniv.edu

M. Mahmud
Department of Computing and Technology, Nottingham Trent University, Clifton Lane, Nottingham NG11 8NS, UK
e-mail: mufti.mahmud@ntu.ac.uk

M. H. Tania
Department of Engineering Science, Institute of Biomedical Engineering, University of Oxford, Headington, Oxford OX3 7DQ, UK
e-mail: marzia.hoquetania@eng.ox.ac.uk

K. C. Santosh and A. Joshi (eds.), *COVID-19: Prediction, Decision-Making, and its Impacts*, Lecture Notes on Data Engineering and Communications Technologies 60, https://doi.org/10.1007/978-981-15-9682-7_10

1 Introduction

Over the last decade, robotics, the Internet of Things (IoTs), and Machine Learning (ML) techniques reached its maturity and intended to use in healthcare applications. The Internet of Healthcare Things (IoHT) integrates IoT and ML models to improve the quality of healthcare services (diagnosis, monitoring, treatment) at an affordable cost [1–4].

The global life expectancy has raised by 5 years with the decease of child death rate, improvement in treating for (non) communicable disease. Besides, the people are aging quickly due to the unhealthy diet, unmanaged lifestyle (smoking, high consumption of alcohol). The World Health Organization (WHO) approximated that some countries have a scarcity of healthcare service providers. A four million health-workers are required to provide acceptable quality healthcare services around the globe [5].

To keep this in mind, the global commercial market segment for the IoT and Robotics is raising at a high pace and intended to be used in the healthcare sector for assisting medical personnel for the monotonous routine task and making the medical procedure safer and less costly for patients [6].

This book chapter is expected to provide an overview of the next generation smart healthcare, precis of robot technology for assisting both doctors/clinicians and patients, design consideration and application (mainly surgery and rehabilitation) of robotics for healthcare services. Besides it also includes the application of robots in screening coronavirus disease (COVID-19), disinfecting hospital premises, assisting in hospital logistics.

The rest of the chapter is organized as follows: Sect. 2 introduced the concept of next-generation smart healthcare architecture; Sect. 3 discussed basics about the robot and its design consideration for the healthcare setting; Sect. 4 explained all the possible application of robots for healthcare/patient care; Sect. 5 outlined the robotic application in pandemics. Finally, the book chapter is concluded in Sect. 6.

2 Next-Generation Smart Healthcare

The IoHT connects peoples (such as doctors, clinicians, medical staff, and patient), medical devices (imaging devices, monitoring devices, etc.), infrastructure (ambulance, pharmacy, etc.) in a hospital and patient in a home using pervasive sensors. The sensor nodes can interact, collect, and exchange data among people, devices, infrastructures. The main aim of IoHT is to ensure a higher quality of experience and performance at an affordable cost.

The IoHT framework contains five layers, namely, Perception, Mist, Fog, Cloud, and Application (see Fig. 1) [7–9]. The inclusion of automated robotic devices in the IoHT makes the framework holistic.

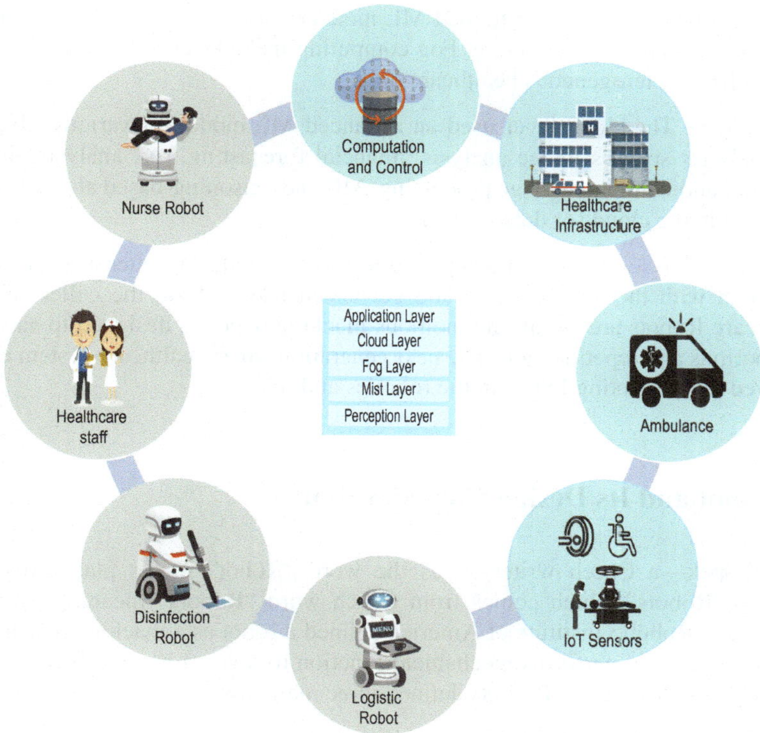

Fig. 1 IoHT integrates robots, healthcare infrastructure, sensors, staff. IoHT layer architecture consists of five layers: perception/sensing layer, mist layer, fog layer, cloud layer, and application/service layer. The fog and cloud layers are responsible for the data analytic, control, and management

Perception/Sensing Layer: In the perceptron layer, the IoT healthcare devices are associated with sensors and actuators. The sensors include physiological sensors (such as temperature sensors, pulse oximeters, blood pressure, and airflow), biosensors (such as Electroencephalography (EEG), Electrocardiography (ECG), and Electromyography (EMG)), and healthcare infrastructure. Along with these sensor data, other data such as laboratory data, imaging data, clinician's advice, patient registration, bill are included in a database called Electronic Health Record (EHR). The perception layer also includes robotic devices connected to the hospital infrastructure.

Mist/Rule Layer: In Mist layer, gateway devices (smartphones, laptops, microcontrollers) collect sensor data and perform real-time rule-based processing and generates an alert. It contains microdata storage and works as a pathway between the physical device and the fog layer. IoT-Fog broker in the Mist layer acts as a mediator and can be configured to manage healthcare sensing data.

Fog Layer: In fog layers, pre-trained ML model is used for data visualization and reduction, and anomaly detection. Fog computing includes ensuring real-time data analysis from heterogeneous healthcare data.

Cloud Layer: The cloud layer used an advanced ML model for various advanced data analytics such as image analysis, financial forecasting, risk analysis, disease detection, and natural language processing. ML and reasoning-based algorithms are employed in the cloud for data analysis.

Application/Service Layer: The application layer provides an interface for people to interact with the infrastructure and get visual insight from the collected data. Healthcare Robots are (semi)-autonomous machine which is designed to carry out the laborious and repetitive job. The next generation smart healthcare system can be deployed by integrating IoT with the robotics and IoT.

3 Robot and Its Design Consideration

Karel Capek—a Czech writer—uses the word "Robot" in his play "Rossum's Universal Robots" which comes from Czech word "Robota" meaning "compulsory labor." Robotic Institute of America defined a robot as a machine which lacks responsiveness but performs mechanical function to assist a human. Issac Asimov (1942) [10] in his series of robots defined three main laws

- **1st Law**: "A robot may not injure a human being, or, through inaction, allow a human being to come to harm."
- **2nd Law**: "A robot must obey the orders given it by human beings except where such orders would conflict with the 1st Law."
- **3rd Law**: "A robot must protect its own existence as long as such protection does not conflict with the 1st or 2nd Law."

Robots are used for hazardous or repetitive job and mainly used by military and space center. With the increasing demand, robots are now being used for healthcare services. In healthcare, the robot can be used to collect physiological data and bio-signal from a patient at the hospital or home and detect anomaly in real time which can be used for personalized care, designing an assistive device for replacing loss function; to collect image/video which can be utilized in image-guided surgery and intervention; to understand human behavior, emotion, and physiological state which can be used for behavioral therapy and rehabilitation. Also, robots can be used in hospitals for wellness promotion, collects samples such as blood or swab from the patient having an infectious disease such as COVID-19, disinfecting places or instruments, and dispense medication and other logistics.

Figure 2 shows capabilities and application area of healthcare robots.

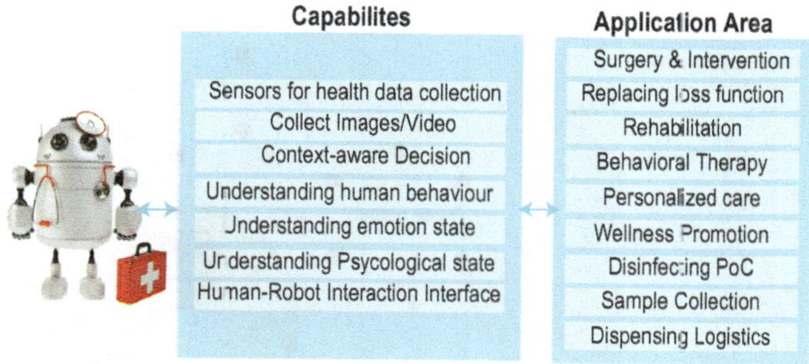

Fig. 2 Capabilities and application area of robots in the healthcare system

4 Robots in Healthcare

The robots are gradually emerging with capabilities to transform the landscape of healthcare with improved accuracy, more precise diagnosis, remote intervention, and augmented human abilities.

4.1 Robots for Surgery

Surgery is a sophisticated discipline ability to treat a plethora of diseases and conditions. Surgical robots—also called cobots—which can assist surgeon or medical experts to perform surgeries. Robot-assisted surgery provides better view of incision via a microscope; reduced pain, discomfort, bloodless, transfusion, and faster recovery via precision surgical procedure. Thus robot-assisted surgery is used in ophthalmic surgery [11], heart surgery [12], knee replacement surgery [13], abdominal surgery [14], etc. Therefore, robotic surgery platforms have found an affluent new market in the medical assistive device industry.

Generally, in robotic surgery, the surgeon operates (finger, wrist, and hand movement of robotic arm) from a computer console, looks at magnified image of surgical site via a 3-D camera and controls robotic arm to create tiny incisions in the patient (Fig. 3).

Table 1 shows surgical robot used in the healthcare setting.

4.2 Rehabilitation and Assistive Robots

Robot for Special Need population: People with neuro, mental, cognitive, and physical disorders are rising every year which increases the demand for designing robots for assisting the special needs pollution. The neuro disabilities include congenital

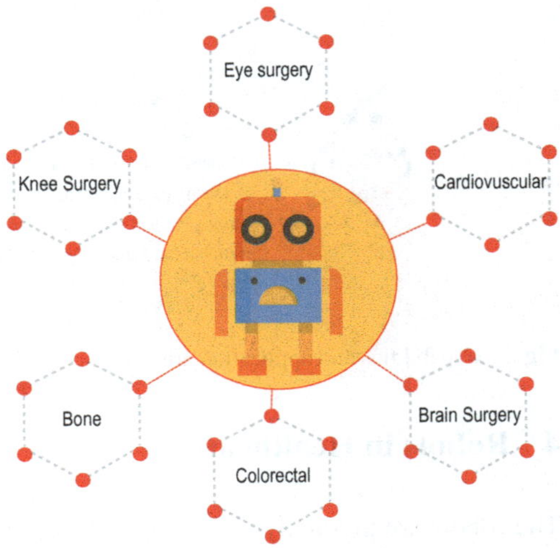

Fig. 3 Surgical area of robots in the smart operating room

Table 1 Surgical robot in healthcare

[15]	Da Vinci	Intuitive	Robotic arm for holding tools; 3-D camera; Stapling
[16]	Mako	Stryker	Joint replacement surgery
[17]	CyberKnife	Accuracy	Radiation therapy; 6-D dynamic motion
[18]	Navio	Smith & Nephew	Image free registration; Robotic-assisted bone preparation; 3-D imaging
[19]	Medtronic	Mazor Robotics	Monitoring patient's health during surgery; Precise cutting; Measuring cutting line
[20]	Auris	Auris Health	Flexible robotic arm for endoscopy; Real-time result on Monarch's bronchoscopy
[21]	Medtronic	Hugo RASH	Cutting; Sealing; Robot-assisted surgery and laparoscopic applications
[22]	Excelsius GPS	Globus Medical	Fiducial marker; 3-D CT scan; Navigated instruments; Position tracker; Drilling capability; Navigated screw guide
[23]	ROSA	Zimmer Biomet	Bone resections capabilities; 360° Imaging of Knee
[24]	Niobe	Stereotaxis	Magnetic navigation; Magnetic maneuverability

such as autism spectrum disorder, brain injury at any stage of the age and neurodegenerative diseases such as Alzheimer, Parkinson, and dementia, these diseases require personalized context aware-long-term assistance. Mental disabilities include anxiety, bipolar/mood, eating, and personality disorder; metal disabilities refer to a neurocognitive disorder. Physical disabilities include visual/hearing loss, chronic fatigue, seizures, a genetic disorder due to the developmental disorder, and disabilities due to injury, illness, and infection. In order to assist physically challenged people, context-aware personalized robotic systems can be used.

Biomedical Robots: Biomedical Robots provide a virtual environment using the knowledge of medical experts and can be utilized in helping the learning (such as disease diagnose or cure) process of surgeons/dentists.

Companion Robot: Alleviation from social isolation and loneliness is an essential reason for social companion robots. Additionally, it can offer assistance beyond emotional support by enhancing the independence among people with special needs. For example, an autonomous bus boarding wheelchair system [25, 26] that can give freedom of movement to wheelchair users by following its companion side by side or in front-behind positions and simultaneously; it has the bus boarding capabilities to detect buses and bus doors with precise measurements of the doorstep's height and width to board and disembark the bus.

Robotic Organ/Bionic prostheses: Robotic assistance can also be served in the form of intelligent prosthetic. Human-made organ artificial robotic organ, a device run by power storage, can be integrated into a human body for replacing the function of the natural organ. For example, bionic prostheses (e.g., arm, leg), neural prostheses (brain), cochlear implant (ear), visual prosthesis (eye), artificial heart, kidney, liver, lung, etc. [27, 28] (Table 2).

Table 2 Various types of robots used for rehabilitation

References	Robot name	Service area
[29]	MIT-Manus	Stroke Patients
[30]	Lokomat	Spinal Cord injury
[25]	TOYOTA-BMR	Smart Wheelchair
[31]	F320	Athletic training and physical therapy
[32]	Ekso	Gait training and neurorehabilitation
[33]	Bioxtreme	Traumatic brain injuries
[34]	Welwalk WW-2000	Lower limb paralysis
[35]	ReoGo-J	Upper limb paralysis

4.3 Acceptability of Robot for Healthcare

Context-aware functionality and capabilities: Robots are autonomous or semi-autonomous systems that are designed for a special function in healthcare to replace human effort. The healthcare robot requires ultra-high precision in executing a specific task at a particular speed. These functionality and capabilities are limited by the evolution of the technology available in the robotic domain and the context. Besides, the healthcare robot requires to be tuned based on the functionality required of an individual, for example, an assistive device designed for a patient cannot be used for another patient, and it must be returned based on the age, sex, and physical strength of that individual [36].

Patient Safety and System's Reliability: Medial robots are paving their pathways to the everyday environment. Thus, separate patient safety standards for professional-service robots (tasks include disinfecting places, surgery, etc.), mo- bile robots (tasks include investigate patient condition, awareness, etc.), collaborative robots (task includes interaction with the patient) are essential to use them in the next generation healthcare setting. A mobile robot moves throughout a workspace and approaching a patient/healthcare stuff who is doing a task that is unrelated to the task of the robot. In such a situation, the task-based risk assessment is required to be investigated [37].

Ethical Perspective: The robot and robotic agent is expected to provide improved patient experience with low cost for healthcare services. Increasing attention toward healthcare robots raises the concern of ethical perspective to be considered in designing and deploying such robots from the perspective of hospital, doctor, medical staff, caregiver/attendee, and patient, socio-cultural lives [38]. The robotic agents are viewed as a tool for assisting healthcare system, thus, the engineer shall consider ethical perspective during the designing and development phase of medical robot and clinicians and medical staffs must be engaged for patient care with the robotic system to achieve social/emotional goal and ethical decision [39].

5 Robots in Pandemics

COVID-19 increased the visibility of robots in hospitals for the daily task in order to reduce transmission of infection in the hospital. The efforts made by the robotic industry to rise to the challenge may forward the market into the mainstream. There is also a projection for the mobile robotics market to grow to USD 23 billion by 2021 [40].

5.1 Robots for COVID-19 Screening

Lowering avoidable and unnecessary physical contacts is one of the key factors that can bring success in managing the coronavirus crisis. The risk of contracting the virus can be significantly reduced for the patient-facing healthcare professionals if advanced robotic screening mechanisms could be in place.

Lifeline Robotics, a spin-out company of the University of Southern Denmark (SDU), has designed and developed to automate the swab testing [41]. The AI-enabled system uses computer vision to correctly identify the region of interest. The automation starts with a patient identification check and ends with safely securing the sample in a container—all the steps can be completed within seven minutes, whereas the core swab takes 25 s. The processing time does not include the sample analysis time, as this robot is not an analysing bot.

The Chinese robot company, Youibot (http://youibot.com/), has rolled-out a multi-purpose robot that can monitor customer's temperatures using infrared cameras during the daytime and disinfect surfaces with the help of UV light in high-traffic areas including hospitals at night. In addition to hospitals in Wuhan, the autonomous indoor robot Aris-K2 of Youibot has already been deployed at Hefei Airport.

5.2 Robots for Disinfecting Hospital

Autonomous bots are often being transformed or adjusted to reassign task such as collaborative robots for machine tending and warehouse rack-stacking are being deployed in the fight against novel coronavirus. Drones originally designed to spray pesticides for agricultural applications have been quickly repurposed to spray disinfectants to fight against COVID-19. DJI is one of the companies who shared the responsibility to disinfect millions of square meters in China [42]. The spraying method entails an efficient discharge of a chlorine or ethyl alcohol-based disinfectant from the air as sanitisation can be carried out 50 times faster than conventional methods. In addition to DJI, other commercial companies such as XAG Technology joined the efforts by China Agricultural Machinery Distribution Association, China Agricultural University Research Centre for Medical Equipment and Application Technology to strengthen the disinfecting program across China with a high standard, as reported by the World Economic Forum [43].

Where DJI is mainly used at public spaces, a Danish company, UVD Robots by Blue Ocean Robotics,[1] sold in more than 40 countries, has been managing Hospital-Acquired Infections (HAI). UV light at wavelengths within 200–280 nm is called UV-C light, is a long-established disinfectant in healthcare settings. The autonomous robot of UVD Robots, consisting thermal cameras and eight bulbs to emit concentrated UV-C ultraviolet light, is capable of destroying bacteria, viruses, and other

[1] http://www.uvd-robots.com/.

harmful microbes by damaging their DNA and RNA, preventing their multiplication. The robot can cost more than fifty thousand pound each.

Another successful example is of HAI is by Xenex,[2] which is widely adopted worldwide. As an US-based company, Xenex managed to deploy its system in hundreds of hospitals in the US, including sites and hospitals operated by the U.S. Department of Defense and Veterans Administration. Another US-based company, GermFalcon, has a solution to disinfect the airplanes.[3]

Despite the surge in demands as well as in sales, the robotic application in the clinical settings needs to be scientifically evaluated to demonstrate the claims made by the companies, which is often missing.

5.3 Robot for COVID-19 Awareness

To prevent the spreading of coronavirus, students in Taiwan built a LEGO robot [44] to encourage school students to wash their hands for hand sanitizing. It's a simple project of robotic hand to hold the sanitizer bottle and act like touch-less faucets with ultrasonic sensor to detect the presence of hands.

Every society is trying to minimizing the spread of COVID-19 virus by maintaining social distance in public places such as a park, bus, and railway station for walkers, runners, and other park visitors to stay several feet away from one another. The Singapore government is using a robotic dog called Spot:2 [45] to ensure that people are using the proper social distance from each which is developed by Boston Dynamics, a Massachusetts-based engineering and robotics company.

Humanoid robots can have an impact on creating social awareness in public places such as the market, and the shop. Kasper [46] is capable of identifying human emotion using pupil's location and gaze pattern that is being used in the USA market places at the entry places of the shop for profiling the shopping habits. Currently, this robot is being utilized for awareness of the people to maintain social distance and giving information on washing hands and coughing etiquette in public places. Another robot developed by Softbank robot, named Pepper [47], capable of detecting masked people, measuring body temperature in the shop, is working in market places to reduce the risk of the virus spreading by reminding people regarding protective measures such as wearing mask, hand washing, and keeping social distance.

5.4 Robots for Assistance in Hospital Logistics

Logistic robots are widely used in industry, warehouse, and manufacturing to automate the storing or moving goods. In near future, smart logistic robots with an

[2]https://www.xenex.com/.

[3]https://www.germfalcon.com/.

integrated infrastructure will roam around the Hospital to move food, lab samples, and other logistics [48].

Unmanned vehicles can reduce the human-contacts that is strictly necessary during the transport cycle of infectious diseases such as COVID-19. Such robots also possess the capability to optimize the delivery time, which can improve the quality of care in the healthcare domain. Utilization of drones for efficient healthcare services is no longer in its infancy, as anticipated. Successful implementation has been already demonstrated in China by commercial entities such as Terra Drone Corporation and Antwork who facilitated the transportation of medical samples from the Xinchang Hospital to the Center for Disease Control and Prevention in Zhejiang. Zipline, a US-based company, has been utilizing drones to deliver vital medical supplies to clinics up to 85 km away in the rural communities in Rwanda and Ghana that reduces a day trip, if conventional means were to use, to 30 min.

Trials have begun in a Scottish island to explore the opportunities for a faster and reliable solution to transport vital medical supplies in hard to reach areas. The drone-based delivery trial is due to run until June 5, 2020 between Lorn and Islands District General Hospital in Oban on Scotland's west coast to the Mull and Iona Community Hospital in Craignure on the Isle of Mull, which can be replicated to other health boards across the UK, if successful [49]. Infrastructure exists to carry out the delivery by-road as well as river taking under an hour, however, such delivery services have been disrupted by the amid pandemic. Thus, a partnership between Skyports and Thales to conduct this trial can not only provide an alternative safer means with less risk of coming in contact with the virus but also can downscale the commuting time to only about 15 min. Similar initiatives have been taken in other parts of the world as well as such as in the outskirts of North Carolina [50].

Although all age groups are at risk of contracting COVID-19, the disease severity could be significantly higher for older people, as indicated by the World Health Organization [5]. Chile has designed a pilot drone program in Zapallar to deliver medication and supplies to isolated elderly people [43]. It can be a two-hour walk from the nearest pharmacy in the hilly locality. Such an initiative has the potential to provide support to the shielded population without exposing a public worker or a member of the family. This program also intends to support the underprivileged who lack personal transportation.

There are hard to reach places, where consumer delivery has been challenging before the amid pandemic. Unprecedented times require unprecedented actions. An example of delivering goods via drones, beyond medical needs that has been expedited due to the coronavirus, is in Anxin's series of semi-isolated islands. Local government in this Chinese county partnered with JD7 to facilitate several drone delivery corridors which resulted in the reduction of hours-long drives with a drone-enabled delivery system under 10 min.

This unprecedented time has taught us the need to learn from each other more than ever. Hence, the World Economic Forum, the World Bank, the International Civil Aviation Organization (ICAO), along with commercial partners have been involved in raising awareness on how to accelerate the use of drones in combating COVID-19 (Fig. 4).

Fig. 4 Various types of robots used during COVID-19; **a** Nurse Robot, **b** Disinfection Robot, and **c** Logistic Robot

Table 3 Some of the popular robots used for fighting against COVID-19

Function	Name	Description	References
Disinfecting places	UVD	UV light to disinfect places	[51]
	S8.2	Contain thermal fogging machine	[52]
	DJI UAV	Drone to disinfect outdoor	[43]
Supply logistic	TIAGo	Supply food	[53]
Sample collection	Life line	Collect throat swab	[41]

Table 3 shown popular commercial robots used for fighting against COVID-19 pandemic.

6 Conclusion

With the increasing demand of IoHT services, the interest of researchers and industries is being pointed toward healthcare robots. In addition, humanoid robotics is evolving firstly in healthcare settings. This book chapter provides an overview of robotic technology and its usability in the next generation healthcare system. Healthcare robots are expected to assist patient care at the hospital and home. Thus, the robotic agent can enhance healthcare experiences by reducing patient care work and strenuous/repetitive manual tasks. The robotic applications can also be used in the management of COVID-19 pandemics. Such applications include collecting the sample from a patient for screening, disinfecting the hospital, supply logistics, and food to the infected patient, collect physiological conditions. However, the long term impact on engaging robots is yet to unfold concerning unintended consequences on human behavior and interaction, inequality at the societal and personal level, privacy and security and above all, singularity of human dominance.

References

1. Afsana F et al (2018) An energy conserving routing scheme for wireless body sensor nanonetwork communication. IEEE Access 6:9186–9200
2. Mahmud M, Kaiser MS, Hussain A (2020) Deep learning in mining biological data. arXiv: 200300108 [cs, q-bio, stat]. abs/2003.00108:1–36. ArXiv: 2003.00108. Available from: http://arxiv.org/abs/2003.00108
3. Kaiser MS et al (2018) Advances in crowd analysis for urban applications through urban event detection. IEEE Trans Intell Transp Syst 19(10):3092–3112
4. Mahmud M, Kaiser MS, Hussain A, Vassanelli S (2018) Applications of deep learning and reinforcement learning to biological data. IEEE Trans Neural Netw Learn Syst 29(6):2063–2079
5. WHO (2020) The world health report 2006—working together for health. WHO. Access date: 11 June 2020. Available from: https://www.who.int/whr/2006/en/
6. Global Commercial Robotics Market: Industry Analysis and forecast 2026. Available from: https://www.maximizemarketresearch.com/market-report/global-commercial-robotics-market/39675/
7. Asif-Ur-Rahman et al (2018) Toward a heterogeneous mist, fog, and cloud-based frame- work for the internet of healthcare things. IEEE Internet Things J 6(3):4049–4062
8. Biswas S et al (2014) Cloud based healthcare application architecture and electronic medical record mining: an integrated approach to improve healthcare system. In: Proceeding ICCIT. IEEE, pp 286–291
9. Mahmud M et al (2018) A brain-inspired trust management model to assure security in a cloud based IoT framework for neuroscience applications. Cognit Comput 10(5):864–873
10. Three Laws of Robotics (2020) Access date: 22 Apr 2020. Available from: https://en.wikipedia.org/w/index.php?title=ThreeLawsofRobotics&oldid=970351529
11. Fine HF, Wei W, Goldman RE, Simaan N (2010) Robot-assisted ophthalmic surgery. Can J Ophthalmol 45(6):581–584
12. Coste-Manière È, Adhami L, Mourgues F, Bantiche O (2004) Optimal planning of robotically assisted heart surgery: first results on the transfer precision in the operating room. Int J Robot Res 23(4–5):539–548
13. Moon YW et al (2012) Comparison of robot-assisted and conventional total knee arthroplasty: a controlled cadaver study using multiparameter quantitative three-dimensional CT assessment of alignment. Comput Aided Surg 17(2):86–95
14. Hanly EJ, Talamini MA (2004) Robotic abdominal surgery. Am J Surg 188(4):19–26
15. da Vinci R (2020) Intuitivel robotic assisted systemsl da Vinci Robot. Access date 22 Aug 2020. Available from: https://www.intuitive.com/en-us/products-and-services/da-vinci/systems
16. Hozack W (2018) Multicentre analysis of outcomes after robotic-arm assisted total knee arthroplasty. In: Orthopaedic Proceedings vol. 100. The British Editorial Society of Bone & Joint Surgery; pp 38–38 (2018)
17. Kurup G (2010) CyberKnife: a new paradigm in radiotherapy. J Med Phys/Assoc Med Phys India 35(2):63
18. Battenberg AK, Netravali NA, Lonner JH (2020) A novel handheld robotic-assisted system for unicompartmental knee arthroplasty: surgical technique and early survivorship. J Robot Surg 14(1):55–60
19. Medtronic Clinical Research (2020) Available from: https://www.medtronic.com/in-en/about/Clinical-Research.html
20. Johnson & Johnson (1986) J&J's Auris touts prelim data from first-in-human study of Monarch platform—mass device. Available from: https://www.massdevice.com/jjs-auris-touts-prelim-data-from-first-in-man-study-of-monarch-platform/
21. Medtronic Surgical Robotics (2015) Available from: https://bit.ly/2EoW5ue
22. Jiang B, Ahmed AK, Zygourakis CC, Kalb S, Zhu AM, Godzik J et al (2018) Pedicle screw accuracy assessment in ExcelsiusGPS§R robotic spine surgery: evaluation of deviation from pre-planned trajectory. Chin Neurosurg J 4(1):1–6

23. Zhang Q et al (2020) Robotic navigation during spine surgery. Expert Rev Med Devices 17(1):27–32
24. Carpi F, Pappone C (2009) Stereotaxis Niobe§R magnetic navigation system for endocardial catheter ablation and gastrointestinal capsule endoscopy. Expert Rev Med Devices 6(5):487–498
25. Al Mamun S, Ali S, Fukuda H, Lam A, Kobayashi Y, Kuno Y (2018) Companion following robotic wheelchair with bus boarding capabilities. In: 2018 joint 7th international conference on informatics, electronics & vision (ICIEV) and 2018 2nd international conference on imaging, vision & pattern recognition (icIVPR). IEEE, pp 174–179
26. Kaiser MS, Chowdhury ZI, Al Mamun S, Hussain A, Mahmud M (2016) A neuro-fuzzy control system based on feature extraction of surface electromyogram signal for solar-powered wheelchair. Cognit Comput 8(5):946–954
27. Gaskill III HV (1990) Intravasular artificial organ. Google Patents. US Patent 4,911,717
28. Aman M, Sporer ME, Gstoettner C, Prahm C, Hofer C, Mayr W et al (2019) Bionic hand as artificial organ: Current status and future perspectives. Artif Organs 43(2):109–118
29. Krebs HI, Ferraro M, Buerger SP, Newbery MJ, Makiyama A, Sandmann M et al (2004) Rehabilitation robotics: pilot trial of a spatial extension for MIT-Manus. J Neuroeng Rehabilit 1(1):5
30. Riener R, Lu¨nenburger L, Maier IC, Colombo G, Dietz V (2010) Locomotor training in subjects with sensori-motor deficits: an overview of the robotic gait orthosis lokomat. J Healthcare Eng 1
31. Prentice WE et al (2004) Rehabilitation techniques for sports medicine and athletic training
32. Kazerooni H, Amundson K, Angold R, Harding N (2014) Exoskeleton and method for controlling a swing leg of the exoskeleton. Google Patents. US Patent 8,801,641
33. Pagliarini L, Lund HH (2016) Redefining robot based technologies for elderly people assistance: a survey. J Robot Networking Artif Life 3(1):28–32
34. Hirano S, Saitoh E, Kagaya H, Sonoda S, Mukaino M, Tsunoda T et al (2018) Wel- walk facilitate early improvement in walking independence of stroke patients with hemiplegia. Annals Phys Rehabilit Med 61:e93
35. Volpe BT, Krebs HI, Hogan N (2003) Robot-aided sensorimotor training in stroke rehabilitation. Adv Neurol 92:429–433
36. Khan A, Anwar Y (2019) Robots in healthcare: a survey. In: Science and information conference. Springer, pp 280–292
37. Kazanzides P (2009) Safety design for medical robots. In: 2009 annual international conference of the ieee engineering in medicine and biology society. IEEE, pp 7208–7211
38. Torresen J (2018) A review of future and ethical perspectives of robotics and AI. Front Robot AI 4:75
39. Westerlund M (2020) An ethical framework for smart robots. Technol Innov Manage Rev 10(1)
40. Intelligence M (2020) Robotics marketl Growth, trends, and forecasts (2020–2025). Available from: https://www.mordorintelligence.com/industry-reports/robotics-market
41. Robotics L (2020) SWAB robotics. Available from: https://www.lifelinerobotics.com
42. DJI (2020) DJI helps fight coronavirus with drones—DJI ViewPoints, DJI Hub. Accessed 03 Jan 2020. Available from: https://content.dji.com/dji-helps-fight-coronavirus-with-drones/
43. Sherwood D (2020) This Chilean community is using drones to help the elderlyl World Economic Forum. Accessed 20 Apr 2020. Available from: https://www.weforum.org/agenda/2020/04/drone-chile-covid19/
44. Everington K. News T, editor (2020) Taiwanese students fight Wuhan virus with robotic Lego alcohol sprayer. Taiwan News. Available from: https://www.taiwannews.com.tw/en/news/3894997
45. He J, Shao J, Sun G, Shao X (2019) Survey of quadruped robots coping strategies in complex situations. Electronics 8(12):14
46. Rossi A, Moros S, Dautenhahn K, Koay KL, Walters ML (2019) Getting to know kaspar: effects of people's awareness of a robot's capabilities on their trust in the robot. In: 2019 28th IEEE international conference on robot and human interactive communication (RO-MAN). IEEE, pp 1–6

47. Robot S (2020) Meet Pepper: the robot built for peoplel SoftBank Robotics. Available from: https://softbankrobotics.com/us/pepper
48. Niechwiadowicz K, Khan Z (2008) Robot based logistics system for hospitals-survey. In: IDT Workshop on interesting results in computer science and engineering
49. Culbertson A. News S, editor (2020) Coronavirus: drones to deliver COVID-19 tests and PPE to Isle of Mull. Sky News. Available from: https://news.sky.com/story/coronavirus-drones-to-deliver-covid-19-tests-and-ppe-to-isle-of-mull-11994656
50. McFarland M (2020) North Carolina hospital turns to drones to aid covid-19 response- CNN. CNN. Available from: https://edition.cnn.com/2020/05/28/tech/drones-covid-19-hospital/index.html
51. UVD. Home—UVD Robots (2020) Available from: http://www.uvd-robots.com/
52. SMP. Spraying robot for unmanned disinfection of large scale open area; 2020. Available from: https://smprobotics.com/products autonomous ugv/ disinfection-spraying-robot/
53. TIAGo (2020) TIAGo—ROBOTS: your guide to the world of robotics. Available from: https://robots.ieee.org/robots/tiago/

COVID-19: A Necessity for Changes and Innovations

Himadri Mukherjee, Ankita Dhar, Sk. Md. Obaidullah, K. C. Santosh, and Kaushik Roy

Abstract The issue of COVID-19 surfaced in late December of 2019. Since then, it is a global threat. One of the major attributes of COVID-19 is the highly infectious nature of the virus. Researchers have been trying to find ways to cure or at least prevent additional spreading. In the literature, we observe developments toward COVID-19 positive case detection with the use of artificial intelligence-driven tools (Santosh in J Med Syst 44:93 [1]). As multitudinal and multimodal data can make a difference in decision-making, there has recently been a trend to put together several datasets of varied sizes over time. Besides, COVID-19 has socio-economic impact across the World. In this chapter, we provide a quick understanding of COVID-19 from both technical innovations (AI-driven tools for prediction and detection) and socio-economic issues. In other words, challenges, innovations and opportunities are discussed in this chapter.

Keywords COVID-19 · AI · Prediction · Decision-making · Multitudinal and multimodal data

---

H. Mukherjee (✉) · A. Dhar · K. Roy
Department of Computer Science, West Bengal State University, Kolkata, India
e-mail: himadrim027@gmail.com

A. Dhar
e-mail: ankita.ankie@gmail.com

K. Roy
e-mail: kaushik.mrg@gmail.com

Sk. Md. Obaidullah
Department of Computer Science and Engineering, Aliah University, Kolkata, India
e-mail: sk.obaidullah@gmail.com

K. C. Santosh
Department of Computer Science, The University of South Dakota, Vermillion, SD, USA
e-mail: santosh.kc@ieee.org

K. C. Santosh and A. Joshi (eds.), *COVID-19: Prediction, Decision-Making, and its Impacts*, Lecture Notes on Data Engineering and Communications Technologies 60, https://doi.org/10.1007/978-981-15-9682-7_11

1 Introduction

The recent outbreak of a Coronavirus in the name of COVID-19 made the entire World not only panicked but people are working tremendously to find a solution to combat this deadly RNA virus. Going back to late December 2019, a large outbreak of a novel coronavirus infection found in Wuhan Province of China.[1,2] Coronaviruses are already known to the human body which is a common cause of cold, cough and other respiratory-related diseases. Since 2003, at least 5 new variants of human coronaviruses have been discovered [2]. To be more specific, SARS (severe acute respiratory syndrome) and MERS (Middle East respiratory syndrome), are two well know coronavirus diseases that have huge mortality rates of 10% and 37%, respectively.[3,4] Till date, COVID-19 affected more than 21,294,845 people across the world with more than 761,779 death cases.[5]

In this chapter, primarily a brief outline of the structure of Coronavirus is presented. This is followed by minute details about disparate COVID-19 Information sharing systems that have been developed by disparate academic institutes and organizations. Some of such sources are discussed herewith. Thereafter different research progress in the avenue of COVID-19 scenario prediction and COVID-19 screening is discussed. This is followed by information regarding disparate datasets that have been put together by researchers to facilitate research in this field. In the penultimate section, the socio-economic impact of COVID-19 is discussed which is followed by the conclusion.

In what follows, let us discuss about the structure of Coronavirus.

2 Structure of Coronavirus

Coronaviruses are spherical in shape and have the ability to alter their morphology, functions or reproductive fashion in respect to environmental conditions. They contain single-stranded (positive-sense) RNA connected to a nucleoprotein within a protein shell surrounding its genetic material. The particles carry club-shaped glycoprotein projections that are in charge of attaching the host cell and also bear the main antigenic epitopes identified by neutralizing antibodies. Most human coronaviruses can be classified into two categories: 229E-like and OC43-like. They both differ

[1] https://www.who.int/docs/default-source/coronaviruse/who-china-joint-mission-on-covid-19-final-report.pdf.

[2] Novel coronavirus—China. https://www.who.int/csr/don/12-january-2020-novel-coronavirus-china/en/ Date: Jan 12, 2020.

[3] Summary of probable SARS cases with onset of illness from 1 November 2002 to 31 July2003. https://www.who.int/csr/sars/country/table2004_04_21/en/.

[4] Middle East respiratory syndrome coronavirus (MERS-CoV). https://www.who.int/emergencies/mers-cov/en/.

[5] https://www.who.int/emergencies/diseases/novel-coronavirus-2019/situation-reports.

in antigenic determinants and culturing requirements. 229E-like coronaviruses can be secluded in human embryonic fibroblast cultures while OC43-like coronaviruses can be secluded or accommodate to growth in unweaned mouse brain. OC43 also have haemagglutinin. The small antigenic cross-reaction between 229E-like and OC43-like can cause independent epidemics of indistinguishable diseases.

All coronaviruses usually evolve in the cytoplasm of infected cells, growing into cytoplasmic vesicles from the endoplasmic reticulum. These vesicles are expelled from the cell within the same period of time and then the cell is destroyed. More details are presented in [2].

Before heading to AI-driven tools for prediction and decision-making (screening), in what follows, we discuss different tracking resources that are freely available.

3 COVID-19 Tracking

Several institutes and organizations had come up with disparate tools for tracking the spread of COVID-19. This had helped researchers to gain valuable insights regarding different aspects of the pandemic. Some of them are mentioned hereafter:

John Hopkins University[6]: It is an interactive map that shows country-wise cases along with different metrics like active cases, incidence rate and hospitalization rate to name a few.

Centers for disease control and prevention[7]: They present disparate details related to COVID-19 outbreak in the thick of number of cases and deaths by jurisdiction, cases and deaths by county and new cases per day.

European Centre for Disease Prevention and Control[8]: They provide COVID-19 situation update on a regular basis. They provide visualizations of their data along with the sum of cases and deaths per country.

World Health Organization[9]: WHO has provided a very interactive and informative dashboard regarding COVID-19 cases. They have presented globally confirmed cases and deaths. They also have presented information of different regions that can be visualized on either weekly or daily basis.

---

[6]https://coronavirus.jhu.edu/map.html.

[7]https://www.cdc.gov/coronavirus/2019-ncov/cases-updates/cases-in-us.html.

[8]https://www.ecdc.europa.eu/en/geographical-distribution-2019-ncov-cases.

[9]https://covid19.who.int/.

4 AI-Driven Tools for COVID-19 Prediction and Screening

One of the most important avenues has been to predict the nature of spread and development of the COVID-19 infection spread across the Globe. Researchers have made use of multitudinous techniques for this purpose [3]. Researchers have mainly adopted three disparate models in the thick of SEIR/SIR models, curve fitting models and agent-based models. However, there are different uncertainties like demographics, test rate, lung and heart-related issues which can cause COVID-19 scenario predictions to deviate from the usual track. The different models barely take into account such uncertainties and hence are not very close to the actual scenario [3]. Li et al. [4] presented an analysis of the transmission process of COVID-19. They made bold predictions regarding the trend of epidemic development in multifarious countries like Italy, South Korea and Iran. Tomar and Gupta [5] presented a data-driven long short term memory-based technique for forecasting of situations. They estimated the number of positive cases of COVID-19 in India for the upcoming 30 days. Sujath et al. [6] also worked on the prediction of COVID-19 situation in India. They used linear regression coupled with multilayer perceptron and vector autoregression. They concluded that a multilayer perceptron produced better prediction results.

Several systems have been proposed for the detection of COVID-19. A large chunk of the systems are based on deep learning which work with either chest X-rays or chest CT-scans. COVID-19 CXR and CT-scan are presented in Figs. 1, respectively. Ozturk et al. [7] used a deep learning-based approach to detect COVID-19 from X-rays. They experimented with over 100 images and reported an accuracy of 98.08%. Mangal et al. [8] presented a system named CovidAID to detect COVID-19 cases from X-rays using deep learning approach. They experimented on a publicly available dataset consisting of over 6 K images and reported an accuracy of 90.5% with 100% sensitivity. Asif et al. [9] presented a deep learning-based approach with convolutional neural networks for COVID-19 identification from chest X-rays. Experiments

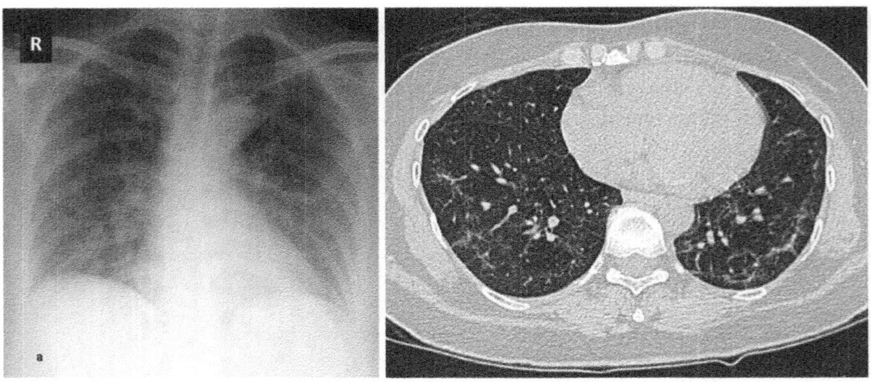

Fig. 1 A COVID-19 infected chest X-ray (left) and chest CT scan (right) https://github.com/ieee8023/covid-chestxray-dataset

were performed with over 3 K images and a validation accuracy of 93% was reported. Das et al. [10] presented a system for screening COVID-19 cases. They experimented with 6 datasets and reported an accuracy of 99.96% with an AUC value if 1.

Walvekar and Shinde [11] used a ResNet50-based technique for identification of COVID-19 cases from chest CTs. Experiments were performed on publicly available data and an accuracy of 96.23% was reported with a sensitivity of 97.15% They also reported precision and F1-scores of 95.60% and 96.37% respectively. Purohit et al. [12] presented a deep learning-based approach for COVID-19 detection. They experimented with publicly available dataset of both CXRs and CTs. They reported accuracies of 98.97% and 95.38% for CXRs and CTs respectively. On applying multi-image augmentation, the CT dataset produced sensitivity and specificity values of 94.78% and 95.98% respectively. In the case of X-rays sensitivity and specificity values of 99.07% and 98.88% were reported respectively. Singh et al. [13] presented a deep learning-based technique for identification of COVID-19 cases from CT images. Experiments were performed on publicly available data and nearly 1.98% better results were proposed using their technique as compared to standard techniques.

5 Publicly Available Datasets

One of the primary requirements for development of any system is the availability of datasets. Researchers have put together datasets of different types to spearhead research in all avenues related to COVID-19. Most of these datasets are changing every day as new data is coming in on a daily basis.[10] is a dataset comprising day level information on COVID-19 affected cases. A COVID-19 testing dataset is available,[11] which can aid to understand and model several aspects in the thick of number of tests per day, tests per confirmed case, etc. CORD-19[12] is an important dataset that consists of over 200,000 scholarly articles related to COVID-19. This has the potential of serving as a source of literature and also influence development of techniques to derive fruitful insights from these articles. The covid-chest X-ray dataset[13] consists of chest X-rays and CT scans of patients with and without COVID-19. It has both lateral ad frontal images of X-rays. Further, the images are of different qualities which is very close to real world conditions. It also consists of images of other diseases like SARS, MERS, pneumonia, etc. This dataset has been widely used by researchers. A CT image dataset of COVID-19 cases is available in.[14] The images are verified by a radiologist. This dataset has also been used by researchers for development of CT-based systems.

---

[10] https://www.kaggle.com/sudalairajkumar/novel-corona-virus-2019-dataset.

[11] https://ourworldindata.org/coronavirus-testing.

[12] https://www.kaggle.com/allen-institute-for-ai/CORD-19-research-challenge.

[13] https://github.com/ieee8023/covid-chestxray-dataset.

[14] https://github.com/UCSD-AI4H/COVID-CT.

6 Socio-Economic Impact and Emotions

The infectious nature and rapid spread of COVID-19 have left a deep mark in humanity. There have been large scale lockdowns all across the globe. This has led to loss in business. Workforce has been lost in almost all economic sectors and plenty of jobs have been lost [14]. People have become more concerned and have developed a very amiable relationship with masks and sanitizers. Street sanitizations have now become a common sight. Almost all of the tourist spots are now closed and people are advised to stay mostly indoors. Though the demand for various commodities and manufactured products has decreased, the demand for medical supplies has increased big time. Moreover, the demand of food products has increased mostly due to stockpiling and panic buying. National and International travel amenities are also now available in an extremely planned way. Academic activities and meetings are mostly being carried out by means of video conferencing. This has brought in a new dimension in academics and the way in which students learn. Most of the scientific conferences have either been cancelled or postponed to later dates. A high number of conferences have shifted to online mode. However, the networking between the attendees has decreased significantly due to this. The much confusion regarding lockdowns has now subsided slightly. The doctors and administration have been working overtime in order to cope up with and tackle the virus.

7 Conclusion

In this chapter, several aspects of COVID-19 are briefly discussed. Here, the basic structure of coronavirus is discussed followed by clinical aspects of COVID-19. A ray of light is cast on some of the available systems for tracking the progress of the pandemic. It is observed that researchers have developed very good and user-friendly systems to bring to light the daily effect of the virus. This has ensured that most people are well aware of the situation. It is followed by a discussion of some of the proposed detection and forecasting systems for COVID-19. Researchers have mostly adhered to deep learning-based techniques for detection of COVID-19 symptoms. Dataset is extremely important for any experimental study. Over time, different datasets have come up to aid in research in numerous ways. Some of them are also outlined in this chapter. This is followed by the impact in the lifestyle of people. The rustics have faced this issue bravely and with caution along with unparallel support from the medical staff and administration. Researchers are still working tirelessly to develop a vaccine for COVID-19 which is expected soon as reports of preliminary results.

References

1. Santosh KC (2020) AI-driven tools for coronavirus outbreak: need of active learning and cross-population train/test models on multitudinal/multimodal data. J Med Syst 44:93
2. Kahn JS, McIntosh K (2005) History and recent advances in coronavirus discovery. Pediatr Infect Dis J 24(11):S223–S227
3. Santosh KC (2020) COVID-19 prediction models and unexploited data. J Med Syst 44(9):1–4
4. Li L, Yang Z, Dang Z, Meng C, Huang J, Meng H, ... Shao Y (2020) Propagation analysis and prediction of the COVID-19. Infect Dis Model 5:282–292
5. Tomar A, Gupta N (2020) Prediction for the spread of COVID-19 in India and effectiveness of preventive measures. Sci Total Environ 138762
6. Sujath R, Chatterjee JM, Hassanien AE (2020) A machine learning forecasting model for COVID-19 pandemic in India. Stoch Environ Res Risk Assess 1
7. Ozturk T, Talo M, Yildirim EA, Baloglu UB, Yildirim O, Acharya UR (2020) Automated detection of COVID-19 cases using deep neural networks with X-ray images. Comput Biol Med 103792
8. Mangal A, Kalia S, Rajgopal H, Rangarajan K, Namboodiri V, Banerjee S, Arora C (2020) CovidAID: COVID-19 detection using chest X-ray. arXiv preprint arXiv:2004.09803.
9. Asif S, Wenhui Y, Jin H, Tao Y, Jinhai S (2020) Classification of COVID-19 from chest X-ray images using deep convolutional neural networks. medRxiv.
10. Das D, Santosh KC, Pal U (2020) Truncated inception net: COVID-19 outbreak screening using chest X-rays. Phys Eng Sci Med 1–11
11. Walvekar S, Shinde D (2020) Detection of COVID-19 from CT images using resnet50. In: Detection of COVID-19 from CT images using resnet50 (May 30, 2020)
12. Purohit K, Kesarwani A, Kisku DR, Dalui M (2020) COVID-19 detection on chest X-ray and CT scan images using multi-image augmented deep learning model. BioRxiv.
13. Singh D, Kumar V, Kaur M (2020) Classification of COVID-19 patients from chest CT images using multi-objective differential evolution–based convolutional neural networks. Eur J Clin Microbiol Infect Dis 1–11
14. Nicola M, Alsafi Z, Sohrabi C, Kerwan A, Al-Jabir A, Iosifidis C et al (2020) The socio-economic implications of the coronavirus pandemic (COVID-19): a review. Int J Surg (London, England) 78:185

Prediction to Service Delivery: AI in Action

Meenakshi S. Arya and S. Prasanna Devi

Abstract When the entire world was abuzz with words like Industry 4.0, Smart cities, Smart World, and innovations and deliberations were being done on how to leverage the latest advances in Artificial Intelligence and Automation to increase productivity, the world got engulfed by an unforeseen pandemic the COVID-19. A sudden surge in demand for Digital Services for Healthcare and monitoring as well as in the field of education has emerged. AI-based system can come to rescue at these times and can significantly aid in processes right from the prediction of the disease to logistics management to delivery of services. A multitude of systems, models, and algorithms are being designed and developed rampantly to cater for this need. The chapter aims to throw light on how this technology is being leveraged with a special emphasis on how AI is revolutionizing Education 4.0.

Keywords Pandemic · Service delivery · RPA models · AI algorithms · Education 4.0

1 Introduction

The event which will go down the annals of history as the most trying times for human beings has brought the entire world to a standstill. However, speaking proverbially "Every dark cloud has a silver lining" and COVID-19 is no exception. When the world began to cripple and economies began to fall, and any human intervention in COVID affected areas started becoming dangerous, the AI systems were brought into action. The time and stage became perfect to exploit the power of this niche technology and numerous devices powered by AI for combating the crisis.

M. S. Arya (✉) · S. P. Devi
Department of CSE, SRM Institute of Science and Technology, Chennai, India
e-mail: raina.arya@gmail.com

S. P. Devi
e-mail: prasannasiva11@gmail.com

K. C. Santosh and A. Joshi (eds.), *COVID-19: Prediction, Decision-Making, and its Impacts*, Lecture Notes on Data Engineering and Communications Technologies 60, https://doi.org/10.1007/978-981-15-9682-7_12

2 Prediction

An artificially intelligent system is capable of predicting the outcomes of any event on the basis of historical data. More the historical data available, better training the model can undergo and accordingly more accurate results it is likely to give. AI has already come into action with AI models like BlueDot being the first ones to identify the emerging risk from the pandemic. Major players in technology including the Tech Giants like Google and Apple are cooperating on contact tracing using AI models. Plethora of coronavirus dashboards showing interactive maps and visuals depicting the virus spread, infection rates and deaths, breakdown of affected and likely to be affected areas, etc., is available online, the most prominent ones being UpCode, NextStrain, John Hopkins University, WHO and Microsoft Bing COVID-19 Tracker dashboards.

The known AI models which were earlier trained for different systems are being re-trained using COVID data to assist in predicting and identifying potentially vulnerable and already infected people. In addition to that, these models help us to anticipate and comprehend the seriousness and geological spread of the virus. The research being conducted at Carnegie Melon University [1] is trying to retrain the models previously trained for normal flu to predict the rise and fall of COVID-19 cases as well. The technique of "nowcasting" uses recent and historical data streams gathered from various sources including Google searches, Twitter activity, and web traffic on the CDC, medical sites, and Wikipedia and feeds them into machine-learning algorithms for predicting the current number of people infected.

In addition to this, models have been designed extending from the traditional rule-based scoring systems to advanced machine learning models (deep learning) and are being utilized by various hospitals across the globe [2]. Epic's deterioration index, which was being earlier used to monitor hospitalized patients, is now being used by dozens of hospitals to predict which Covid-19 patients will become critically ill and hence cater for the essential resources required to manage these critical cases [3].

A model using machine learning and standard epidemiology has been developed by a team of engineers at MIT. This model is built to determine the efficacy of quarantine measures using the available data and feeds this data to a neural network which helps better predict the spread of the virus [4].

3 Logistics Management

The wholesale, retail and supply chain sectors across the globe have been shaken by the COVID-19 crisis. Long periods of lockdowns and lone periods of Quarantine have made people buy and hoard things that they might not even need. But the fear of unknown is gripping everyone and hence the supply chains are under extreme stress. Delays in Shipment, shortage of skilled manpower labour and disruptions to the aviation industry have toppled global logistics. Although the supply chain resilience has been improved by the tech industry, with the spread of the virus, new technologies are gaining power. Supply chain leaders are looking at AI and smart analytics to ensure flexibility in times of crisis and are aiming at faster adoption of the same to predict what products are going to be in demand and when. Researchers have proposed various AI-based models that try to establish a correlation between the logistic variables relevant to a specific sub-problem and the corresponding supply chain costs [5]. Certain areas which can most definitely be aided with AI-based solutions for the management of logistics are.

3.1 Supply Chain Management

Capturing the need for demand and supply through various online platforms and applying Machine Learning (ML) for Supply Chain Planning (SCP) can play an extremely critical role in the delivery of products. Leveraging the potential of artificially intelligent tools that can facilitate in building concrete plans is the key to the current situation. ML models can revolutionize the way decisions are made as far as forecasting of inventory, demand and supply is concerned. It will provide a foresight into the future and thus avert any kind of shortage of goods and services. The industry can focus on using Robotic Process Automation (RPA) and chatbots for Operational Procurement (speaking to suppliers during trivial conversations, processing and forwarding of purchase orders, generation and processing of various compliance and governance reports), Inventory Management Automation (keeping an eye on inventory levels, sending notifications and automatic reordering when stock levels fall below a threshold, predicting the optimal inventory levels by taking into account the historical data and outlining the patterns in demand, restocking of inventory), Order processing and procurement (selection of the product, payment processing and order placement confirmation) and Communication(opening the email, making sense of what the customer needs, logging into the ERP system, to communicating the exact status, self-triggering emails and text messages to the stakeholders for communication).

These tools can aid in extracting the requisite and relevant data from the company database, processing of the transactions from the electronic payment gateways and sending or confirming the placement of orders through automated emails and text messages. Some of the commonly used RPA tools are Blue prism, Automation AnyWhere, UiPath, etc. RPA in Supply Chain, along with the power of AI-ML, can enable organizations to eradicate the possibility of human intervention (which has become the need of the hour) and forecast demands and hence be more prepared to accommodate the unexpected rises in demand.

3.2 *Autonomous Vehicles for Logistics and Shipping Management*

As this pandemic has forced people to go into extended periods of self-isolation, quarantining as well as work from home, it has resulted in a huge increase in the demand of essentials like food, groceries, household items and even medical supplies such as masks or personal protection equipment. The governments as well as the people want these goods and supplies to be delivered to their doorsteps. Due to this, the logistic infrastructure is heavily stressed worldwide as currently there appears to be a huge strain on global supply chains ranging from medical supplies to household goods.

Unmanned Delivery Vehicles with AI-assisted systems can come as a big rescue and reduce the risk of spreading infection. For example, in China, popular companies like JD.com, Meituan and Keenon Robotics are utilizing autonomous logistic vehicle to deliver goods, fresh vegetables and food so as to reach people in hospitals and quarantine zones in more than 40 cities. Though the mobility and logistic sectors are under significant impact by the COVID-19, the pandemic may be "The Silver Lining in the cloud" to try out the new technology and accelerate the deployment of such vehicles. Non- traditional Players like Google, IBM, Apple. Uber Technologies and even amazon are also heavily investing in making autonomous vehicles a reality. At the present phase of technology development, self-driving long-haul trucks can be used for automation of the middle mile. TuSimple, which was over the last year transporting parcels for United Parcel Service (UPS) between Phoenix and Tucson, Arizona, included the new route connecting Phoenix with El Paso, Texas during the month of March.

4 Service Delivery

Covid-19 not just led to the disruptions to the daily lives of common people, it off-boarded the complete service industry, be it aviation, travel or tourism, hospitality or education. With travel and education being the ones to bear the biggest brunt. Universities, Colleges and Schools were one of the first organizations to be closed due to more chances of biggest disruption. Growth in adoption of Artificial Intelligence (AI) powered education has paved a way to uninterrupted continuation of education during the Covid-19 pandemic lockdown. The term Industry 4.0 was coined when manufacturing industries started adopting technology, similarly the term Education 4.0 refers to this period wherein education sector embraced technology to keep the show going. The application of AI in Education 4.0 has seen a phenomenal growth and it is evident that the AI-based systems have complemented the teachers, students and administrators in sustaining education anywhere and anytime, including the times of lockdown.

4.1 Best Practices of Education 4.0 During the Pandemic

Many schools and colleges have rebooted the education during Covid-19 by making use of the technology and shifting towards online teaching and learning process. For the students in remote areas who are unable to get the benefits of technology through live sessions, the lectures were archived in Google classroom so that students can use it for learning at a later point in time.

With the current generation students geared up with education 4.0, the technology is leveraged to reach students during this Covid 19 breakdown and for higher education institutions, this implies how it can be used to reach students for continuing the teaching, learning, examination and administration process.

Some of the best practices of implementing education 4.0 are given below and a few best practices implemented in the present generation educational institutions are given in Fig. 1.

1. The process of learning in education 4.0 has seen a shift from typical classroom learning to 'learning on the go', which facilitates gaining knowledge while travel, at home, at park and at anyplace, anytime. The challenges in extending this anytime, anywhere education during the Covid-19 includes extending the practice of software-based programmes and circuit-based laboratory courses that are made possible by virtual labs.
2. Flexible delivery of classes still continues uninterrupted even during the lockdown period with the online delivery of classes conducted by the faculties. This enables the students to gain knowledge even from their parent institution and they also have access to learning from global tutors as well.
3. Mentoring of students becomes vital in this digital age wherein students have access to most of the jungled information and the teacher's role becomes vital.

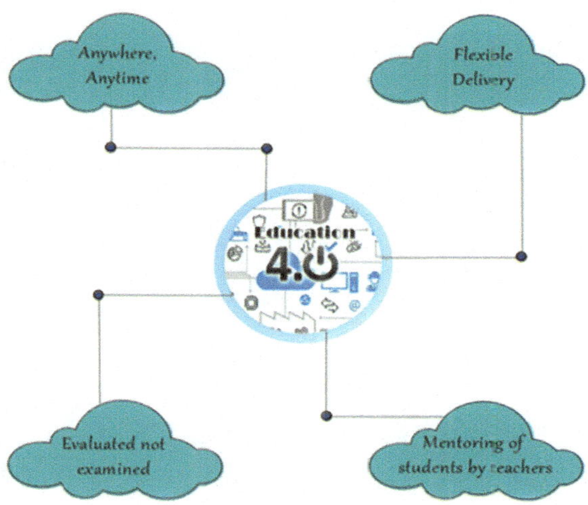

Fig. 1 Best practices of AI for education 4.0

They are responsible in curating their learning content and providing instant feedback on the learning process of the student and to quantify their levels of learning. This also enables the mentor to give feedback on a student's successful learning path among a larger group thus makes evidence-based learning foolproof.
4. To make the students industry ready, they must not be assessed by the traditional question and answers methods, but tested on the application of their knowledge is of utmost importance.

The above best practices of Education 4.0 has helped the education sector continue its services uninterrupted during the pandemic Covid-19 outbreak.

4.2 Pivotal Role of AI in Education 4.0

A wide range of software sources deploying AI/ML have been implemented across educational institutions. A few use cases of the same are given in Table 1.

AI methods used in the above use cases are classification, regression, clustering, structured prediction, robotic process automation and natural language processing.

It is evident that AI has revolutionized the education 4.0 in terms of promoting transparency, potential in removing bias and easing the uninterrupted flow of education. The rise of AI-based use cases in education 4.0 has challenged the conventional education and has contributed in large to detect, monitor and correct the bias in the educational process wherever possible. Though the pace of development of AI-based expert systems for educational use is accelerating, the adoption of all these sophisticated use cases in the educational institutions is still very slow.

Table 1 AI-based use cases in education 4.0

AI/ML-based Use Cases	Departments	Description	Predominant use of AI/ML algorithms	AI/ML-based use cases	Departments
Facial recognition system	Hostel, Examination, Academics attendance management	To recognize students/outsiders entering the class/hostel premises; Authorize students taking up online examinations	Use of vector representation to match an identity of University personal whose identity is stored in the database	Facial recognition system	Hostel, Examination, Academics attendance management
Chatbots	Admissions, Enquiries in administration	To handle queries related to admissions and to ease the onboarding of new batch of students to the campus	Text classification using Natural language processing and classification algorithms	Chatbots	Admissions, Enquiries in administration
Processing of complaints	All departments	Processing of complaints	The complaints (academic/non-academic) are processed using NLP, categorized, prioritized, trends are identified and sent to respective department head to ensure timely response to every complaint registered	Processing of complaints	All departments
Assessment and behavioural management	Academics	Performs the assessment and behavioural management with minimal human intervention	Deep learning algorithms	Assessment and behavioural management	Academics

References

1. https://www.technologyreview.com/2020/03/13/905313/cdc-cmu-forecasts-coronavirus-spread/
2. https://www.bmj.com/content/369/bmj.m1328
3. https://www.statnews.com/2020/04/24/coronavirus-hospitals-use-ai-to-predict-patient-decline-before-knowing-it-works/
4. https://news.mit.edu/2020/new-model-quantifies-impact-quarantine-measures-covid-19-spread-04164.
5. Bruzzone A, Orsoni A (2003) AI and simulation-based techniques for the assessment of supply chain logistic performance. In: 36th annual simulation symposium. Orlando, FL, USA, pp 154–164

COVID-19 Impacts Construction Industry: Now, then and Future

Soumi Majumder and Debasish Biswas

Abstract The construction industry is one of the most important industries for national development in the world. It is an unorganized sector and most of the time human-driven; a large number of people are working in this sector. In the pandemic of COVID-19 most of the construction sites are being halted due to fear about the infection of Coronavirus. The projects are already delayed in relation to completion and handover. The developers are not facing the cost escalation risk only, also afraid of the spreading of COVID-19 in projects. The model of Work Health and Safety (WHS) laws says that it is the duty of the employers to take care of the health and safety of their workers in the workplace. In the building and construction industry where workers work closely together, there is a high risk of exposure to COVID-19. During this epidemic situation, all the employers and constructors should implement the control measures to minimize the spread of COVID-19 and provide a safe work environment to the workers. In this study, we are highlighting the impact of novel Coronavirus in the construction industry associated with risk assessment and how to implement the safety measures for the workers during and post pandemic.

Keywords Construction · Workers · COVID-19 · Coronavirus · Safety

1 Introduction

The rapid growth of novel Coronavirus has created an alarming health crisis all over the world. Apart from the human impact, the situation generated the impact on commercial activity throughout the globe. As the virus has no border it spreads continuously. The epidemic has turned the global economy into a recession that means the economy has started shrinking and generating no growth. In the US, it is

S. Majumder (✉) · D. Biswas
Department of Business Administration, Vidyasagar University, Midnapore, West Bengal, India
e-mail: majumdersoumihr@gmail.com

D. Biswas
e-mail: debasish762010@yahoo.com

K. C. Santosh and A. Joshi (eds.), *COVID-19: Prediction, Decision-Making, and its Impacts*, Lecture Notes on Data Engineering and Communications Technologies 60, https://doi.org/10.1007/978-981-15-9682-7_13

seen that millions of people have filed the unemployment benefit for this disruption of COVID-19. As per the report of IMF (International Monetary Fund) in many countries the manufacturing output is going to be diminished and shows a fall in external demand as well as domestic demand. The nationwide lockdown creates a fear of no source of earning daily wages into the workers. Thus, migrant laborers were going back to their home towns. The darkness of construction sector got down after the lockdown is lifted. The impact will be manifold in the construction industry due to this pandemic.

The construction sector in India is a development sector. It creates more investment opportunities to increase the national income of the country. This is an unorganized sector and huge labor-intensive. Principle companies, contractors, subcontractors, consultancy all have specific roles to play towards the smooth running of this sector. In 2011–12, the industry had contributed 670,778 crores (US$ 131 billion estimated) to the national GDP with a share of 8.2%. 65% of the total investment in construction comes under the infrastructure of the county. Real estate sector under construction is very much recognized. It is expected that the real estate market will be grown up to Rs. 65,000 crores by 2040 from Rs. 12,000 crores (US$ 1.72 billion) in 2019. It is also expected that the real estate sector will contribute 13% of the country's GDP by 2025. Research has revealed that the real estate sector in India will be increased by 19.5% CAGR by 2028.

India is not the only country to face the predicament in the construction sector for this Covid-19 pandemic. According to the World Bank report on global economic prospect India's gross domestic product (GDP) to be contracted by 3.2% in 2020–21. It is expected that there can be a moderate recovery to 3.1% growth in 2021–22. This says that the GDP of the year 2021–22 will be less than it was in the years 2019–20. In 2018–19 construction had a share of 8% in GVA (Gross Value Added) but as per PLFS (Periodic Labour Force Survey) its employment share was 12% in 2018–19. On the other hand financial services, real estate, and professional services, the GVA share was 22% in 2018–19. The employment share of the construction sector was only 3.4%. It gives the view that construction is a more labor-intensive sector than finance [1].

Due to this COVID-19 pandemic, the investment in construction-related projects has been reduced in the range of 13–30% that will have a significant impact on Gross Value Added (GVA) and employment in this sector. Construction-related GVA is expected to reduce between 15 and 34% and employment between 11 and 25%, respectively. On account of this pandemic, construction sector is expected to face a reduction in both supply and demand simultaneously. The sector is driven by infrastructure projects to a large scale, it is expected that there will be a severe hit by the current levels of uncertainty, loss of income, dismal business, and consumer sentiments as well as the preservation of government funds toward management of COVID-19 [2].

Finally, a fall in the productivity or output of construction sector causing the further shrinking of the overall economic activity. In a post-crisis reality for economic sustainability the construction industry needs to maintain the masses employed, enhance quality of living, and meet project timelines and budgets.

The consequences like reverse migration, disruption of the supply chain, and others make the hindrance to meet the obligations under the construction and engineering contracts [3] during lock down period. The halted construction projects need to reopen with the help of health and safety norms established by the labor acts. The employers and constructors must follow the labor laws related to health and safety to keep the work continuous in post lockdown era [4]. It is well known that the construction industry is huge labor-intensive and the project participants are multicultural, multi-location, multi-disciplinary, and multi-organizational. Therefore, employers should give attention to preserve them by providing a safe work environment. During and after this epidemic, COVID-19 risk assessment of the construction projects is mandatory, and based on the evaluation vivid precautions need to be taken by all the eminent persons who are doing business in construction.

In this study, the prime focus is to highlight the various aspects of health and safety in the construction sector during the global pandemic COVID-19. In Sect. 2, the impacts of COVID-19 in the construction industry are reported. In Sect. 3, risk assessment of the mentioned industry has been discussed. In Sect. 4, safety measures for Coronavirus for the workers are reported. Future construction industry technologies and discussions are mentioned in Sect. 5 and Sect. 6, respectively. Finally, Sect. 7 is the conclusion section.

2 Impacts of COVID-19 in Construction Sector

The impact of the COVID-19 pandemic is very detrimental and a poor impact has been made on the labor market, supply of materials, company liquidity, project delivery, key cost components on construction projects, and so on. Due to the lockdown situation, all sites are being closed across the Globe. People are in-home quarantine for the wellbeing of their health and safety. Many countries like Italy, China, and others face a sharp decrease in the production sector. Contractors and employers who depend on Chinese made goods, materials, and equipment are facing problems like shortage of construction materials, higher cost of such materials, and quipment that lead to slower project completion, moreover more projects have been canceled due to this situation [5].

The worldwide impact of coronavirus in the construction sector has created a poor economic structure; countries infrastructure development is suffering a loss. In India, as per KPMG (Klynveld Peat Marwick Goerdeller) report, it is shown that the overall impact of a novel coronavirus in the construction sector has been estimated near about Rs. 30,000 crore per day. This reduces the investment to the construction-related projects by 13–30% and it creates a significant impact on employment as well as Gross Value added. Again KPMG (a well-known global network of professional firms providing Audit, Tax, and Advisory services) has given an estimation that the cost of skilled workers is expected to rise by 20–25% while semi-skilled and unskilled workers are expected to increase by 10–15%. Based on geographical area and spreading of coronavirus the under-development projects are taking a severe hit with a minimum delay of two to three months. In India as per CREDAI (Confederation of Real Estate Developers Associations of India), there were around 20,000 ongoing projects, before the lockdown. The 68 days lockdown started from March 24, 2020 to May 31, 2020 has created a huge lack in labor supply as all migrated laborers returned to their villages. It was estimated around 6 lakhs workers moved on to their villages and near about 10 lakhs workers were stuck in the relief camp across the country [6].

In this COVID-19 pandemic, this large labor force and their health and safety should be highlighted by the side of the eminent constructors. When the laborers or workers will be coming together to restart their work after reopening the site spreading of COVID-19 is a great risk involved in this sector. The huge spread of coronavirus in the construction sites resulting shutdown of the work immediately. It is not a good sign for the industry progress. Therefore, risk assessment is also an important task of the employers. On the basis of that, they should take the safety measures for all the working personnel in the industry.

3 Risk Assessment

The current and lasting impact of the COVID-19 pandemic has been created a whole new set of risks for every construction project. It is the responsibility of the owners and contractors to identify and manage the risk with this changing scenario of the city due to this epidemic. The risk is the result of halting the project in the construction sector. In the wake of the coronavirus pandemic whenever management will plan and construct a project, they should consider some of the inevitable risks like financial impacts of the pandemic, site safety including workers and others, security of the site, labor shortages, and disruptions in supply chains and so on [7]. The temporary shutdowns lead to unanticipated project delays, governmental orders and permit delays, and reduce crew size with social distancing. The impact of COVID-19 is the same for the construction employees, owners, contractors, and suppliers like the general population. There is no difference between the general population and construction workers for facing these consequences. In every construction site, the owners must provide the physical well-being and safety for all project team members, stakeholders, participants and they must follow the safety guidelines and recommendations which has been proposed by the government authorities and healthcare professionals. There are three types of risk associated with construction projects such as completion risk, commercial risk, and contractual risk [8]. Completion risk includes, many projects are delayed and disrupted due to COVID-19 pandemic. Due to the lockdown situation and tight labor market projects are already struggling to complete tasks on time. COVID-19 has created supply chain disruptions, funding restrictions, and cash-flow concerns which lead to rescheduled and extended of the critical activities. The commercial risk includes extended performance costs, commodity price swings, labor-cost escalation, and higher interest payments. If the handover dates of the project are delayed owners must be faced the higher cost relating to internal project management cost, cost of third-party construction managers and consultants, etc. These delays are the result of an increase in financing cost, developer cost, and management fees. The contractual risk is concerned when the delays, disruption with commercial risk will be giving pressure on contracts and allotting the party to mitigate such risk. From the Contractors viewpoint, it will be saying that they are not responsible for delays as a COVID-19 scenario is unforeseeable and out of the contractor's control [9]. Under these circumstances such contracts allow the contractors to extend the time of project completion and some contracts also allow contractors to recover the increased performance cost.

As per Occupational Safety and Health Administration (OSHA), the job task has four risk exposure levels, they are low-risk level, medium risk level, high-risk level, and very high-risk level [10]. Lower risk level includes jobs that do not require any contact with the people who are suspected of being infected by COVID-19. Examples of lower exposure risk jobs are (i) remote workers (working from home during the epidemic), (ii) manufacturing industry workers who do not have close contact with customers or public, (iii) health workers with telemedicine services, etc.

Medium risk level jobs including the close or frequent contact with the people who may be infected or the people who are not aware or suspected of having COVID-19. Examples are the people who may have frequent interactions with travelers returning from international locations with widespread COVID-19 transmissions and the people who may have contact with the general public like some high-volume retail settings. The third level is high exposure risk level; jobs that are highly suspected with sources of SARS-CoV-2 are included in this category. The construction site workers, contractors, subcontractors, and health care delivery staff and support staff who deliver services to COVID-19 patients are coming under this high-risk zone.

The fourth risk zone is a very high-risk level, in this case there are high potentialities for exposure, people who have high contact with the suspected people or diseased people, or have the interactions with the people who are coming from the containment zone. The construction laborers are coming from different areas so the chances of being infected by them in the site are very high. With them, other construction workers get infected and it can be spread all over the area. Apart from the health workers such as doctors, nurses, emergency medical technicians, etc. are countable here.

We know the construction sector is labor-intensive and it has unique nature due to its complexity. In this sector workers cannot do work from home as it's not possible for the workers to manage the site from sitting at home. When it comes to reopening the site a huge risk factor is involved [11]. Many people like project managers, contractors, dealers, clients, suppliers, supervisors, and labors will be coming together to do the work at the site. Therefore, chances of contamination are very high. As per OSHA guidelines high and very high-risk levels are considered in the construction sector under the section of risk assessment.

4 Safety Management for Restarting Work After Post Lockdown at Site

World Health Organization is researching with the global experts, partners, and governments to find out the cause of rapidly spreading of Coronavirus and providing the necessary advice on control measures to make the people healthy and safe. As per the Guidelines of WHO industrialists should take all necessary preventive and protective measures for workers to minimize the occupational health and safety risk. It provides the information and instruction on usage of PPE (Personal Protective Equipment) and also giving refresher training on infection prevention and control (IPC). All the construction employers, employees, contractors need to follow the released guidance regarding COVID-19 exposure prevention, preparedness, and response. The prevention of workers from the Coronavirus and what protective measures should be taken at job sites with proper disinfecting work practices are discussed in this section [10]. The following are some guidelines for the health and safety of the construction workers which need to be maintained after reopening the sites.

World Health Organization is researching with the global experts, partners, and governments to find out the cause of rapidly spreading of Coronavirus and providing the necessary advice on control measures to make the people healthy and safe. All the construction employers, employees, contractors need to follow the released guidance regarding COVID-19 exposure prevention, preparedness, and response, the prevention of workers from the coronavirus, and what protective measures should be taken at job sites with proper disinfecting work practices [12]. The following are some guidelines for the health and safety of the construction workers which need to be maintained after reopening the sites.

4.1 Guidelines on Work Restart

During the post lockdown phase daily health safety meeting with a briefing session in the morning must be arranged to ensure social distancing norms. During this course of action, the safety officer must be communicated with the workers about health and safety guidelines and necessary updates. To disseminate the information all necessary arrangements for public announcements should be made. The records of all workers at the site including photo identity cards should be maintained. Construction workers should go outside from the site for their necessity items by wearing a face mask after informing the supervisor. Outside workers will not be allowed to stay at the site without following the proper instructions and procedures. In this case, large gathering or meetings should be avoided and also should maintain a minimum of 3 ft distance from persons. Depending on the size two fourth of the total persons should allow traveling either in lift or hoist at the site. Moreover, the usage of the staircase should be increased to maintain the situation.

4.2 Guidelines on the Entry of Construction Site

At the entrance of the site, congestion should be avoided. For reducing the number of workers at workplace, different shifts of work and different areas should be arranged. People who will be handling materials that are coming from the outside they need to be worn hand gloves. Reusable equipment should be cleaned properly. It is mandatory for all the vehicles and machinery which will be entering into the premise that must be disinfected by using the spray. The construction materials need to be untouched for one day after arriving at the site and then workers can use it.

4.3 Guidelines on Labor Protection

In this case, a mandatory thermal scanning for everyone should require for checking fever or body temperature during entry and exit time. If any individual leaves the site and re-enters during the shift re-screening will be done before re-entry into the worksite. Another important measure for the workers is to use masks while working at the site and while not wearing the mask they should cover mouth and nose with tissues in case of cough and sneeze.

4.4 Guidelines On-Site Hygiene

The belongings of the workers like food, water bottles, mobile phones, utensils, etc., should not be shared with others during work time. All the workers need to wash their hands with soap and water for at least 40 s. If hand washing is not possible then hand sanitizer with >70% alcohol should be used. Apart from these spitting in common are must be prohibited and may be punishable with heavy fines. The common sitting arrangements should be removed and food must be consumed at designated areas only to ensure social distancing. The usage of toilets and bathrooms should be done with maintaining social distancing. Gathering and crowding must be avoided at these spots. The handles of equipment and tools that are shared should be disinfected before using. In the case of waste management, no-touch garbage bins with biodegradable garbage bags need to be used at all common access areas along with proper sanitization [13]. With the help of the toolbox talk method, it should be communicated to the workers that they must not touch their eyes, nose, or mouth with unwashed hands during working hours.

4.5 Guidelines on Labor Camp

In the workers, a camp minimum of two or three rooms should be kept as isolation wards. Visitors should not be allowed in the camp. In labor hutment area cleaning of toilets, bathrooms, dining area, and general area can be made regularly. Apart from that de-sanitization of the total camp must be done at frequent intervals. When they will be out of rooms minimum of 6 ft distancing should maintain. If any workers feel any discomfort or symptoms related to COVID 19, they must inform the camp supervisor. In this case, the special concern will be taken by arranging the isolation rooms and proper observation procedures. If conditions of the workers will not be improved within 3 or 4 days it's the responsibility of contractors and employers to send the diseased person to the govt. hospitals for further treatment Employers need to arrange necessities like vegetables, groceries, etc. for the workers to avoid crowding [14].

4.6 Guidelines on Contractors and Staffs

During post lockdown, after reopening of construction site employers should start the projects with 50% staff strength and divide the staff based on their departments. A disinfection tunnel must make at entrants, also must keep the thermal scanning machine for knowing the body temperature. All staffs, contractors, managers must wear a face mask while working. It is mandatory for all construction workers, engineering staff, and others to wash and sanitize their hands before entering and exiting the premises. Sufficient numbers of hand soaps or sanitizers must be stored at the site location. Only 50% of engineering staff should be allowed to travel at the site by private vehicles. After reopening the site, the nonessential visitors from the head office, consultants, and others are strictly banned to visit sites. The entire construction site including sit office, labor camp, toilets, canteens, pathways, entry, and exit gates will be disinfected daily. The housekeeping team with the necessary equipment must be kept in this regard. Appropriate signage with safety practices at the construction site should be maintained in the local language or using that language which is understood by all. The hospitals or the clinics that are authorized to treat COVID 19 patients must be identified and regarding list should be displayed at the site all the time [15].

5 Future Construction Industry Technologies

The COVID-19 outbreak [16, 17] will surely change company policies, work culture, and also increase the use of automatic machines in the construction sector. The clients will surely sift from the real estate industry to various diversified industries like e-commerce, artificial intelligence (AI) automation, logistics, etc. AI will take a significant role in global construction market analysis (competitive landscape and detailed information on vendors), revenue, and forecasting (component, service model, and development model, vertical and geographical analysis) and growth. AI will also take an important role to predict cost overrun of a project (based on size, type of contract, competency level of risk mitigation, automation) [18]. Moreover, upcoming trends and changes in customer behaviors can also be predicted by AI. Besides these, the use of cloud computing will help in mobility and allow users to access relevant records and real-time monitoring [19]. Companies may opt for contextual and/or scripted (or hybrid) chatbots to save time and money. Unmanned Aerial Vehicle (UAV) drone supported with artificial intelligence will monitor construction sites.

It is expecting that the use of prefabricated construction, 3D printing (additive manufacturing), use of augmented reality/virtualization, use of big data and analytics, use of wireless monitoring and connected equipment, 3D Scanning, photogrammetry, etc., will significantly increase in this industry.

6 Discussions

In the construction industry, every employer and constructor should have the obligation to protect the workers from injury and hazards in the workplace as per the regulations of the Occupational Safety and Health Act (OSHA). In this global pandemic COVID-19, the health and safety of workers must be the top concern of the employers. During this post lockdown period, all the parties of the construction sector should provide an increased focus on the health and safety of the workers to keep job sites open [20]. Before the continuance of construction site work, there must be a review of risk assessment is needed. It includes not only the financial risk but also the spreading risk of the coronavirus among the staff or workers. Effective and corrective guidance should be followed for managing the risk. If the guidance does satisfy no further work should take place. Employers should keep in mind that risk can be generated from the virus directly and risk is also generated indirectly that is a huge change will take place in the work practices and what will be the impacts. In this changing work environment, it's not predicted what impact will be created on the economy by these work practices and what will be the effects on staffing levels, availability of equipment, and activity of the third-party contractors or consultants. In the case of revising risk assessment and method statement, these things must be considered.

Once the risks have been identified, control measures can take easily for reopening the sites. The workers must be trained and provided sufficient information regarding COVID-19 to manage those risks. The Coronavirus Act, 2020 helps the government to impose restrictions on the public and industries and create the offence in relation to not obeying the restrictions. The Management of health and safety at Work Regulations, 1999 applies to all the employers to assess and manage health and safety risks and to set out the mechanism for it. The objective of those regulations is to plan, organize, control, and monitor health and safety [21]. Therefore, for the wellbeing of the workers from the side of the employers, the control measures must be maintained, monitored, and properly supervised. In the context of the coronavirus and restart the job of construction sites careful considerations must be taken and implemented in all aspects. If it is not done the work cannot be carried out safely and the country will face more difficulties.

7 Conclusion

The epidemic disease Coronavirus first occurred in Wuhan, China, and then created a worldwide impact in a very short time. The World Health Organization (WHO) declared this novel Coronavirus as pandemic on March 11, 2020. In our country, the effects of this epidemic have been tried to decrease by taking some preventive measures such as travel prohibition, closure of schools, colleges, shopping malls, theaters, workplaces, quarantines, home-office practices, a curfew of citizens above the age of 65 and so on. There was no exception in the case of the construction industry. When the concern comes to the reopening of the construction sites every employer should take care of their employees or workers as per the Constitution and the Labour Code No. 4857. The most inevitable responsibility of the employers according to Code No. 6331 is to take necessary measures relating to occupational health and safety. According to article 4 of the code, employers have some obligations to ensure the health and safety of the employees such as prevention of occupational risk, providing necessary training on account of changing circumstances, monitoring and checking the measures, carrying out the risk assessment, ensuring employees capabilities regarding health and safety, taking appropriate measures in the area of life-threatening and special hazards. Human resources are the most critical resources in every organization. There is a very famous term that is 'Health is Wealth'. Therefore, by providing good health and safety to them the organizations can make their wealth in the near future.

References

1. Economic impact of Covid-19 pandemic to vary in sectors. https://www.hindustantimes.com/india-news/economic-impact-of-covid-19-pandemic-to-vary-in-sectors/story-DIWjwnBZoON7ZUvgSMSFOL.html. Accessed 23 June 20
2. COVID-19 :assessment of economic impact on construction sector in India. https://home.kpmg/content/dam/kpmg/in/pdf/2020/05/covid-19-assessment-economic-impact-construction-sector.pdf?. Accessed 23 June 20
3. Subramani T, Lordsonmillar R (2014) Safety management analysis in construction industry. Int J Eng Res Appl 4(6):117–120
4. Zhao T, Kazemi SE, Liu W, Zhang M (2018) The last mile: safety management implementation in construction sites. Advances in civil engineering. https://www.hindawi.com/journals/ace/2018/4901707/
5. Rowlinson S (ed) (2004) Construction safety management systems. Routledge.
6. COVID-19 impact:construction project hit as workers keep away. https://economictimes.indiatimes.com/industry/services/property-/-cstruction/covid-19-impact-construction-projects-hit-as-workers-keep-away/articleshow/74738820.cms?from=mdr. Accessed 1 June 2020
7. Identifying and managing construction risks during the Coronavirus pandemic. https://www.gouldratner.com/publication/identifying-and-managing-construction-risks-during-the-coronavirus-pandemic. Accessed 1 June 2020
8. COVID-19 risk for construction owners. https://advisory.kpmg.us/articles/2020/covid-19-risks-for-construction.html. Accessed 1 June 2020
9. Neziris ON, Topali E, Papazoglou IA (2012) Occupational risk of building construction. Reliab Eng Syst Saf 105:36–46
10. Choi HH, Cho HN, Seo JW (2004) Risk assessment methodology for underground construction projects. J Constr Eng Manag 130(2):258–272
11. The effects of Coronavirus (Covid-19) on occupational health and safety and an evaluation within the scope of work accidents. https://www.lexology.com/library/detail.aspx?g=40aa95b3-3508-4576-a2c2-9899b5f8be07. Accessed 1 June 2020
12. Kelly TP, McDermid JA (1997) Safety case construction and reuse using patterns. In: Safe Comp 97. Springer, London, pp 55–69
13. Gillen M, Kools S, McCall C, Sum J, Moulden K (2004) Construction managers' perceptions of construction safety practices in small and large firms: a qualitative investigation. Work 23(3):233–243
14. COVID-19: Occupational Health and Safety. https://www.osha.gov/SLTC/covid-19/hazardrecognition.html. Accessed 1 June 2020
15. COVID-19 information for workplaces. https://www.safeworkaustralia.gov.au/covid-19-information-workplaces. Accessed 1 June 2020
16. Santosh KC (2020) AI-driven tools for coronavirus outbreak: need of active learning and cross-population train/test models on multitudinal/multimodal data. J Med Syst 44:93. https://doi.org/10.1007/s10916-020-01562-1
17. Fong SJ, Dey N, Chaki J (2020) Artificial intelligence for coronavirus outbreak. Springer, Singapore
18. Lertpalangsunti N, Chan CW (1998) An architectural framework for the construction of hybrid intelligent forecasting systems: application for electricity demand prediction. Eng Appl Artif Intell 11(4):549–565
19. Kaklauskas A, Zavadskas EK, Trinkunas V (2007) A multiple criteria decision support on-line system for construction. Eng Appl Artif Intell 20(2):163–175
20. Coronavirus-construction sector facing daily loss of Rs. 30,000 crore investments in projects to fall 13–30%: KPMG. https://www.moneycontrol.com/news/real-estate-2/coronavirus-construction-sector-facing-daily-loss-of-rs-30000-crore-investments-in-projects-to-fall-13-30-kpmg-5243761.html. Accessed 1 June 2020
21. Banaitiene N, Banaitis A (2012) Risk management in construction projects. In: Banaitiene N (ed) Risk management—current issues and challenges, pp 429–448

COVID-19 on Air Quality Index (AQI): A Necessary Evil?

Ankit Chaudhary, Vedika Gupta, Nikita Jain, and K. C. Santosh

Abstract The disastrous effect of novel coronavirus has become a matter of concern for human health since December 2019. To counteract the spread of the disease, the many countries' governments-imposed movement restrictions in different approaches. Retarding growth in various sectors had turned out to be a negative repercussion of the imposed lockdown. On the contrary, isolation practices became climate favorable. Improved air quality indices have been observed in many regions due to a halt on constant air polluting activities. In this chapter, we present an analysis of variation in air quality indices of different countries: United States, Brazil, India, Australia, China, and Taiwan.

1 Introduction

The entire world is tackling the unprecedented and severe challenges by the rapid spread of COVID-19. This infectious disease had put humankind in danger. In response to this global crisis, many nations across the world had declared regulations to restrict people's movements to follow social distancing and isolation practices. As a consequence, many countries observed a tremendous downturn in all three

A. Chaudhary · V. Gupta · N. Jain
Department of Computer Science and Engineering, Bharati Vidyapeeth's College of Engineering, Delhi, India
e-mail: ankitchaudhary3010@gmail.com

V. Gupta
e-mail: vedika.gupta@bharatividyapeeth.edu

N. Jain
e-mail: nikita.jain@bharatividyapeeth.edu

K. C. Santosh (✉)
Department of Computer Science, University of South Dakota, 414 E Clark St, Vermillion, SD 57069, USA
e-mail: santosh.kc@usd.edu

K. C. Santosh and A. Joshi (eds.), *COVID-19: Prediction, Decision-Making, and its Impacts*, Lecture Notes on Data Engineering and Communications Technologies 60, https://doi.org/10.1007/978-981-15-9682-7_14

sectors of the economy due to travel constraints. Services like education, information technology, telecommunication, and medical were the least affected.

In contrast, services like construction, transport, travel and tourism recorded a retarding growth, resulting in an economic recession in the world. Besides these unfavorable and negative impacts, lockdown imposition and mobility restrictions proved to be a blessing for nature. This crisis had brought a significant break and relief to the earth from consistent pollution-causing activities. The biosphere had rejuvenated in the lockdown period. Cleaner air, less contaminated water bodies, and low noise pollution are positive impacts due to mobility constraints. Improved air quality in both rural and urban areas is one of the favorable changes that the climate has gone through. A significant decline in air pollution is due to the less emissions of toxic gases from industries, vehicle exhausts, power plants, and forest fires. Limited operations in essential commodities industries remain continued following safety measures. However, most industries and manufacturing units were shut down, which resulted in a decline in the release of significant air pollutants-particulate matter, sulfur, and nitrogen oxides. Also, emissions of gases such as Carbon Monoxide and Sulphur Dioxide have witnessed a reduction due to lesser road and sky traffic. The Air Quality Index (AQI) decreased in many countries due to the restrictions imposed on day-to-day activities and brought environmental benefits.

In this chapter, the impact on the AQI of various countries due to COVID-19 pandemic imposed lockdown is analyzed and discussed. Section 2 presents different studies and investigations conducted made towards AQI analysis during the pandemic. Section 3 puts forth the visualization of the lockdown effect on AQI of various countries. Section 4 reflects upon the analysis visualized in the chapter concerning the impact of AQI during the COVID-19 pandemic.

2 Related Works

The positive implications of lockdowns on air quality have become a subject of interest for researchers around the world. This section discusses the summarized overview of the existing analysis on variation in air pollution, environment, and climatic conditions.

A significant contribution by [1] represents the effects on air quality in March in five metropolitan cities of India, i.e., Delhi, Kolkata, Mumbai, Chennai, and Hyderabad. The concentration of Particulate Matter 2.5 (PM2.5) and Nitrogen Dioxide in the air have been analyzed with HYSPLIT back trajectory and compared with the year 2019. Zoran et al. [2] have discussed the influence of Particulate Matter on COVID-19 cases in Milan, Italy, during the pre-lockdown and the lockdown period. They have observed the parameters like wind speed, air temperature, humidity, and concluded that the spread of COVID-19 would not be controlled in warm conditions. Agarwal et al. [3] have compared the air quality status of cities of India and China during pre-lockdown and lockdown. The analysis was done based on two pollutants, i.e., Nitrogen Dioxide and PM2.5. The results showed that a decrease in Nitrogen Dioxide was more rapid as compared to PM2.5. Another contribution by [4] identified the relationship between the climatic conditions and the COVID-19 cases in New South Wales. The analysis was done on the data consisting of daily rainfall and relative humidity and relative temperature from 9 a.m. to 3 p.m. from February 12 to March 31. Results have shown that temperature and relative humidity affect the transmission of the disease. Studies in [5] have shown that there are no significant changes observed in air pollution in New York City from January 2020 to May 2020. While concentrations of PM2.5 and Nitrogen Dioxide decreased, the magnitude was comparable to those of previous years. No improvement was reported in air quality due to New York City lockdown. In [6], the authors discussed the fruitful impact of lockdown on the environment taking India as a case study. There was a reduction in air, noise, and water pollution during the lockdown in India. Concentrations of air and water pollutants were taken into consideration. Considering PM2.5 as a significant pollutant, Rodríguez-Urrego and Rodríguez-Urrego [7] highlighted the decrease in air pollution in different capital cities of the world. The cities of the continent of Asia were given a major focus by contrasting their pre- and during quarantine times. The average reduction in the concentration of PM2.5 was 12%. In [8], reduction in Nitrogen Dioxide levels in cities of Spain, i.e., Barcelona and Madrid, were observed to be 50 and 62%, respectively, in March. Monthly average concentrations of Nitrogen Dioxide were compared from the previous years 2018 and 2019. Moreover, the contribution of traffic, city, and country transports to declined Nitrogen Dioxide levels in Barcelona and Madrid were taken into consideration. Comparing the 40 cities worldwide, [9] discusses the changes in concentration of PM2.5, PM10, Nitrogen Dioxide, Sulphur Dioxide, Carbon Monoxide, and Ozone from February and March for years 2019 and 2020. Compared with the previous year, PM2.5 decreased in 17 cities in February and 14 cities in March. The analysis shown by [10] depicts that ozone levels went up in the city Rio de Janeiro, Brazil, due to a decrease in Nitrogen Dioxide.

In this chapter, a thorough analysis of the variation in the air quality of various countries, which differ in coronavirus cases and lockdown implementations is discussed.

3 Air Quality Index and Its Variation in Lockdown

Air Quality Index is a numerical scale to determine the healthiness or quality of the air on a day-to-day basis. A higher AQI score indicates a more hazardous and toxic nature of air. AQI is computed by taking into account the concentrations of five air pollutants—Particulate Matter (PM2.5/PM10), Ground-level Ozone (O_3), Nitrogen Dioxide (NO_2), Carbon Monoxide (CO), and Sulphur Dioxide (SO_2). These pollutants are briefly discussed as follows:

I. *Particulate Matter (PM2.5/PM10)*
Particulate Matter refers to the mixture of solid and liquid particles (particularly smoke and dust) suspended in the air. PM2.5 are fine particles with a diameter of less than 2.5 μm, and on the other hand, PM10 are coarse particles with a diameter of less than 10 μm. Due to its very minute size, these particles can enter into the lungs and can cause heart and respiratory diseases like bronchitis or asthma. Harmful emissions from vehicle exhausts, industries, forest fires, and incomplete combustion are some of the primary sources of particle pollution in the air.

II. *Nitrogen Dioxide (NO_2)*
Nitrogen Dioxide gas is reddish-brown in colour and has a pungent odor. It is one of the primary air pollutants in the atmosphere, which is formed during the combustion of fuels in vehicles and industries. Oxides of Nitrogen (NO_x) react to form photochemical smog, acid rain, and other air pollutants like particulate matter and Ozone. Nitrogen oxides can cause negative impacts on human health (respiratory infections) as well as crop yields.

III. *Ground-level Ozone (O_3)*
Ozone can be divided into two types—Stratospheric Ozone and Ground-level Ozone. Stratospheric Ozone protects living organisms from the harsh effects of Ultraviolet (UV) rays. In contrast, Ground-level Ozone is considered as a bad Ozone. It is formed by the chemical reaction between oxides of Nitrogen (NO_x) and volatile organic compounds (VOCs) in the presence of sunlight. Ground-level Ozone has an adverse effect on human health, especially children and adults. Coughing, breathing problems, lung infections, and increased risk of death among patients suffering from heart and lung disease are some of the significant health issues due to increased levels of bad Ozone.

IV. *Carbon Monoxide (CO)*
Carbon Monoxide, a poisonous gas, is produced by the incomplete combustion of fossil fuels in vehicles, industries, and fires. Breathing Carbon Monoxide gas reduces Oxygen (O_2) supply to various organs in the human body by combining with haemoglobin and causes dizziness, headache, unconsciousness, and increased chances of heart diseases.

V. *Sulphur Dioxide (SO_2)*
Sulphur dioxide is a colorless and toxic gas with a suffocating smell. It is formed during the combustion of sulphur-containing fossil fuels, smelting of mineral ores of Aluminium, Copper, and emissions from volcanic eruptions. Along with Nitrogen Dioxide, it contributes to the formation of acid rain. It causes tract infections, coughing, irritation in eyes, and mucus secretion.

The objective of the AQI is to make the public aware of the extent of air pollution or contamination in their surrounding atmosphere or any other region. The AQI values can be classified into six categories based upon their impact on health, as shown in Fig. 1.

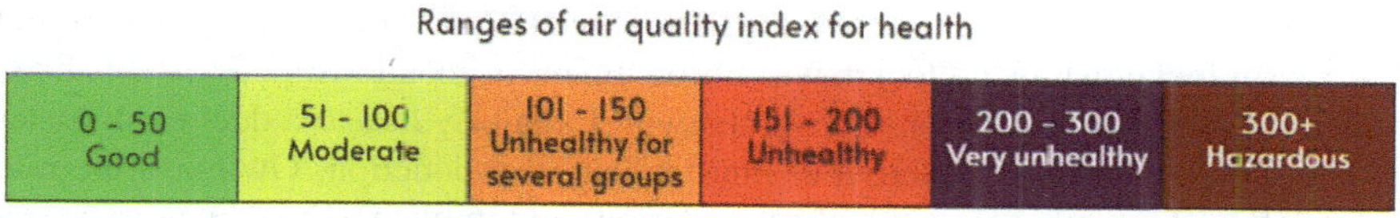

Fig. 1 AQI classification based on effects on human health

3.1 Effect on Air Quality of Different Countries in COVID-19 Crisis

On observing the high spread of novel coronavirus, the government bodies in many nations across the world had imposed curfews, emergency lockdown, and different mobility restrictions. People followed 'stay-at-home' rules and social distancing measures. Borders of many countries were entry restricted. Many ongoing activities either got paused or slowed down during the COVID-19 pandemic situation. The three sectors agriculture, industrial, and service, witnessed a major decline in their operations. Considering a smaller number of transportation services used by the people, the release of harmful emissions of Nitrogen Dioxide, Carbon Monoxide, and Particulate Matter from vehicle exhausts in the air decreased. Uncommonly, private transport on roads in urban areas got reduced in number. Only a few vehicles for unavoidable tasks got permission for plying on the road. The services of electric powered metro trains came to a halt in countries like India. Public transportation services, including buses, taxis, airplanes, and passenger ships were discontinued. Another prominent source of air quality degradation is the discharge of poisonous and toxic gases from industries and power plants. Many industrial hubs and centres were all shut down due to the enforcement of lockdown. Only the production of essential items- food and pharmaceutical products continued at the same rate. Smelting of Sulphur containing metals- Aluminium, Cobalt, and Iron was halted in mineral refining and metal extracting activities, which limit the emissions of gas. Manufacturing and production of non-essential commodities (rubber, plastics, and other electronic equipment) were either stopped or reduced at a higher rate. Electric-powered trains and other organizations heavily rely on high powered electric supply. Shutting down of such institutions depreciated the demand of electrical supply from coal-fired power plants, causing less release of toxic emissions in the atmosphere. Lowering of industrial activities involving the burning of fossil fuels, discharge of untreated gas or harmful by-products into the air, had resulted in improved air quality in many cities during the global pandemic. In addition to these direct consequences, air-polluting activities like- deforestation, smoking, and forest fires reduced to some extent, hence, contributing to better air quality.

Improved air pollution in many countries is due to the different approaches and methods practiced by the nations to follow social distancing measures. These restrictions varied from country to country, depending upon the spread of disease. Countries (United States, India) with high infection rates imposed complete and partial lockdowns, whereas some least affected countries (China, Taiwan) either imposed short-term lockdown or no lockdown. Enforcement of lockdown periods enhanced the air quality in many nations across the world, majorly due to a decline in transport services, construction activities, and industrial production. Owing to the rate of COVID-19 spread, different lockdown periods and implemented strategies, seven countries have been considered for this study for the purpose of visualizing the trends in AQI variation. The analysis of changes observed in AQI values of several countries are discussed as follows:

I. *United States*

In the United States, Los Angeles, Denver, Oklahoma, and Tucson have reported a high incidence of infection with coronavirus. In contrast, only little spread has been reported in North Dakota, South Dakota, and Wyoming counties. In late March 2020, many state governments in the US declared 'stay-at-home' orders leading to shutting down of industries and subsequent reduction of harmful and toxic emissions. Figure 2 shows the visualization of the variation in the monthly average concentration of major air pollutants in cities of the United States. The overall AQI of the United States started declining since February 2020.

Further, the levels of all the contaminants except ground-level Ozone dipped in February and March 2020. Emissions of Carbon Monoxide and Nitrogen Dioxide dropped at a much higher rate from the beginning of February 2020 due to reduced transport usage and industry shutdown. The average concentration of Nitrogen Dioxide gas in Los Angeles decreased around 13 and 50% in February and March. Unlike all other pollutants, ground-level Ozone increased due to the presence of low nitrogen dioxide in winters. As seen in the visualization shown, AQI slightly

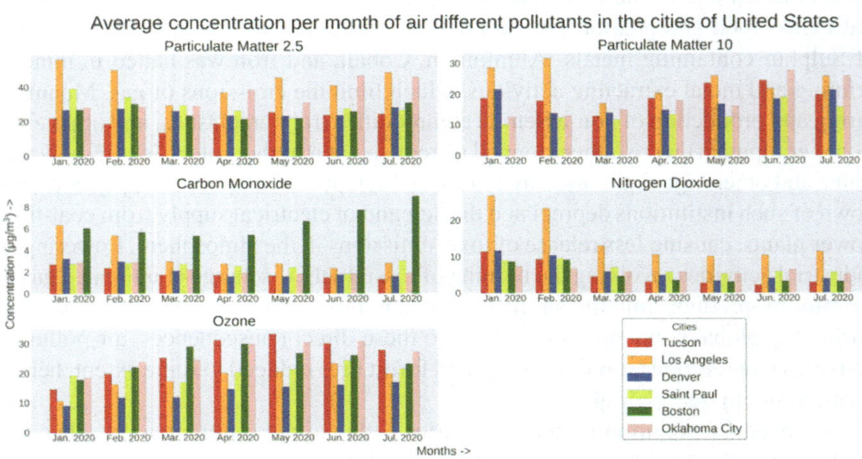

Fig. 2 Variation in air pollutants concentration from January 2020 to July 2020 in the cities of the United States

increased from May 2020 in the cities of the United States due to the reopening of retail stores, restaurants, and places of worship.

II. *Brazil*

A declaration of partial lockdown by the Brazilian government was made on March 24, 2020, which permitted only essential businesses to resume while ensuring safety measures. Operations for public transport were allowed for limited hours because of which emissions of Particulate Matter and Nitrogen Oxide had started rising in March and April, specifically in the regions of São Paulo and São José dos Campos. Also, deforestation and forest fires increased by 20% in Amazon rain forests in the year 2020, which raised the air pollution levels in the cities of Brazil at an alarming rate. Inferring from Fig. 3, concentrations of major air pollutants in Vitoria city decreased to some extent. Average concentration of Sulphur Dioxide in Vitoria declined by 52% in April 2020 as compared to January in the same year.

III. *India*

Following the successful 'Janta Curfew' on March 22, 2020, the Indian government declared a nationwide lockdown on March 24, 2020, for 21 days. As there was no control over the number of rising cases, this lockdown was followed by three more lockdown phases till May 31, 2020, to prevent the spread of coronavirus. Amongst the thirty-five Indian states, Shillong witnessed the least number of COVID-19 cases followed by Bhopal and Kolkata, the cities, as mentioned in Fig. 4. Different mobility restrictions were imposed in all the states. Public transportation services like metro rails, inter-state bus services, and railway trains were shut down in India, resulting in low AQI in cities. As inferred from Fig. 4, the concentration of major air pollutants

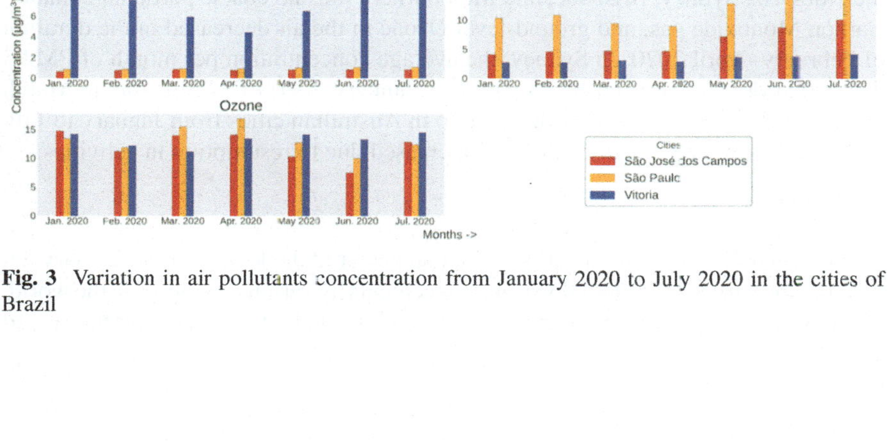

Fig. 3 Variation in air pollutants concentration from January 2020 to July 2020 in the cities of Brazil

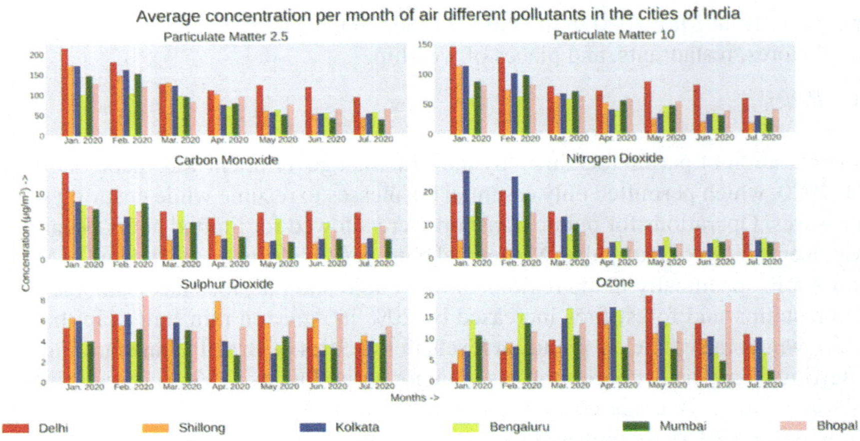

Fig. 4 Variation in air pollutants concentration from January 2020 to July 2020 in the cities of India

dropped by a large number during the lockdown period. Levels of PM2.5 and PM10 in the air were gradually reducing every month. Low emissions of Carbon Monoxide and Sulphur Dioxide were observed in Shillong and Mumbai. A fall in the concentrations of Nitrogen Dioxide in Kolkata and Mumbai regions is because of less demand for ships for foreign trade. Ground-level Ozone was increasing in all the cities from January 2020 to April 2020. Despite the lockdown period, the air quality is still improving in the unlock periods in cities of India.

IV. *Australia*

Australia recorded a lesser number of COVID-19 cases (around 22 k, till August 13, 2020) as compared to countries like the United States, Brazil, and India. Speculating the rapid spread of this disease in advance, borders of Australia were completely closed in February 2020. Flights from other countries China, Italy, United States, were restricted. By the end of March 2020, different lockdown restrictions were imposed in various regions of Australia. Figure 5 depicts a significant change in the air quality of the cities viz. Sydney, Brisbane, and Melbourne. Fine and coarse particulate matter, Carbon Monoxide gas, and ground-level Ozone in the air decreased in the duration of February–April 2020. In Sydney, the average concentration per month of PM2.5 descended drastically from 62.48 $\mu g/m^3$ in January 2020 to 17.3 $\mu g/m^3$ in March 2020. Levels of Nitrogen Dioxide went up in Australian cities from January to July 2020. Following the lockdown, PM2.5 increased due to resumption in activities.

V. *China*

China, where the coronavirus originated, had declared the lockdown on January 23, which is the earliest of all lockdown announcements by various countries in the world. Most of the ongoing activities and services in China halted to counteract the spread

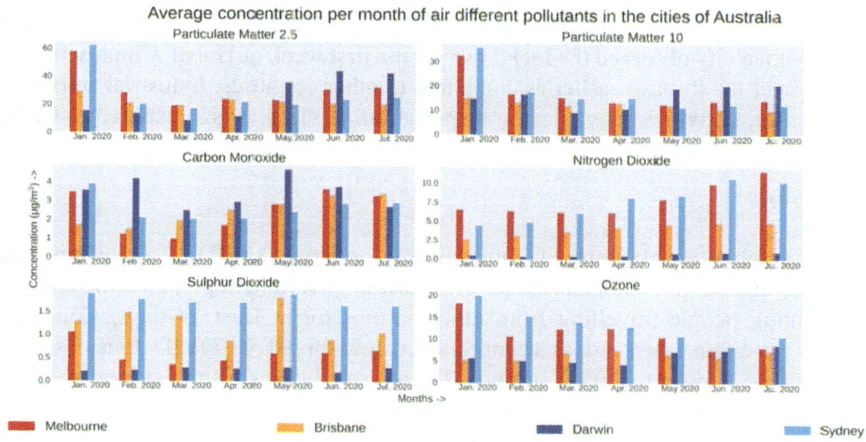

Fig. 5 Variation in air pollutants concentration from January 2020 to July 2020 in the cities of Australia

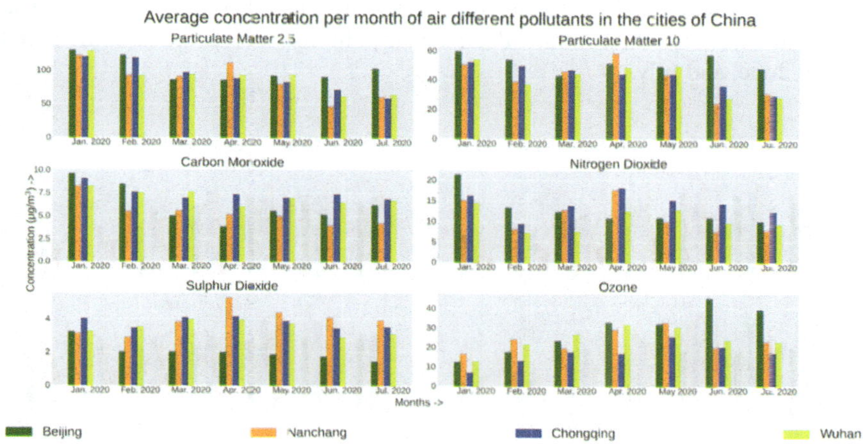

Fig. 6 Variation in air pollutants concentration from January 2020 to July 2020 in the cities of China

of disease. As a consequence, air pollution in the country reduced to a certain extent. The monthly average concentrations of Particulate Matter and Carbon Monoxide in the air improved in Beijing; Fig. 5 shows the trend in the major air pollutants in cities of China during the COVID-19 pandemic. Nanchang, Chongqing, and Wuhan, and on the other hand, the amount of bad-ozone in the air gradually increased. The minimum concentration of Carbon Monoxide in Beijing was recorded to be 1.9 $\mu g/m^3$ in February. Sulphur Dioxide in the areas of Nanchang and Wuhan went up in the lockdown due to ongoing industrial activities. Following social distancing measures smartly, lockdowns in China ended around late March in most of the cities while Wuhan city observed the lockdown till the first week of Hubei. China achieved control over the disease earlier as compared to other countries. Industrial activities, construction activities as well as transportation services, were restarted, causing pollution levels to rise as before.

VI. *Taiwan*

Being a neighbouring country of China, awareness about COVID-19 alarmed people about the disease from January 2020. The Taiwan government prepared the country by isolating people travelling from other nations for at least 14 days. Country's borders were shut down and, as a consequence, low spread of COVID-19 is observed in the cities. Taiwan recorded around 477 confirmed cases till the second week of August. The nation never declared a complete lockdown in the country. Although social gaps were maintained in the public. Hotels, restaurants, and health and beauty care stores were opened. Industrial operations were carried on. People were supposed to maintain distance in the transport. Due to these ongoing activities, air pollution in the cities of Taiwan did not decline significantly. As shown in Fig. 7, the amount of major air contaminants in Taitung City, Taichung, and other cities increased from January to April. On the contrary, declined air pollution was recorded in the month of May, June, and July.

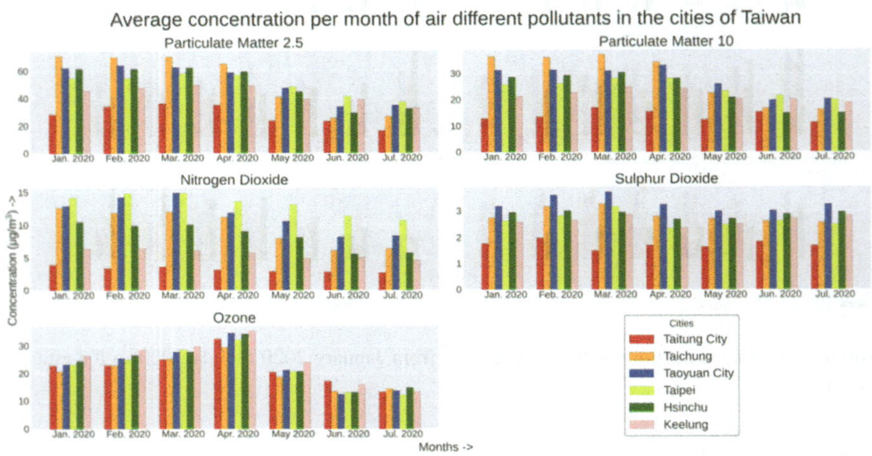

Fig. 7 Variation in air pollutants concentration from January 2020 to July 2020 in the cities of Taiwan

4 Reflections

Due to the rapid spread of COVID-19, many countries declared lockdowns in several phases, which had seized air quality impacting activities, thereby reducing the AQI levels. Starting from late March 2020, India and the United States observed a complete lockdown in the country. Concentrations of particulate matter, Nitrogen Dioxide, and Carbon Monoxide decreased in most parts of India and the United States. In contrast, ground-level Ozone increased due to a decrease in Nitrogen Dioxide. On the other hand, Australia and Brazil imposed a partial lockdown. Australia got a reasonable control over the spread of the disease; thereby, low AQI was observed in Australia in March and April. AQI in Brazil deteriorated due to the fires in Amazon rain forests. Following the smart practices by China, lockdown ended early at the end of March in major cities. A decrease in PM2.5, Carbon Monoxide and Nitrogen Dioxide was recorded due to the increment in ground-level Ozone in many cities. Whereas, Taiwan was alerted by the rapid spread of disease and had a good command against the transmission of the disease in January and February. The country didn't enforce a lockdown; instead reduced very few operations, which didn't reduce air pollution. The lockdown imposition had become favourable and fruitful for the environment. Low AQI values in many countries have been evident. This made government bodies and institutions assured that a significant change could be expected by imposing lockdowns on a regular basis.

References

1. Singh RP, Chauhan A (2020) Impact of lockdown on air quality in India during COVID-19 pandemic. Air Qual Atmosp Health 1–8
2. Zoran MA, Savastru RS, Savastru DM, Tautan MN (2020) Assessing the relationship between surface levels of PM2. 5 and PM10 particulate matter impact on COVID-19 in Milan, Italy. Sci Total Environ 139825
3. Agarwal A, Kaushik A, Kumar S, Mishra RK (2020) Comparative study on air quality status in Indian and Chinese cities before and during the COVID-19 lockdown period. Air Qual Atmosp Health 1–12
4. Ward MP, Xiao S, Zhang Z (2020) The role of climate during the COVID-19 epidemic in New South Wales, Australia. Transbound Emerg Dis 1–5. https://doi.org/10.1111/tbed.13631
5. Le Quéré C, Jackson RB, Jones MW, Smith AJ, Abernethy S, Andrew RM, ... Friedlingstein P (2020) Temporary reduction in daily global CO_2 emissions during the COVID-19 forced confinement. Nat Climate Change 1–7
6. Arora S, Bhaukhandi KD, Mishra PK (2020) Coronavirus lockdown helped the environment to bounce back. Sci Total Environ 140573
7. Rodríguez-Urrego D, Rodríguez-Urrego L (2020) Air quality during the COVID-19: PM2. 5 analysis in the 50 most polluted capital cities in the world. Environ Pollution 115042
8. Baldasano JM (2020) COVID-19 lockdown effects on air quality by NO_2 in the cities of Barcelona and Madrid (Spain). Sci Total Environ 140353
9. Shrestha AM, Shrestha UB, Sharma R, Bhattarai S, Tran HNT, Rupakheti M (2020) Lockdown caused by COVID-19 pandemic reduces air pollution in cities worldwide
10. Siciliano B, Dantas G, da Silva CM, Arbilla G (2020) Increased ozone levels during the COVID-19 lockdown: Analysis for the city of Rio de Janeiro. Brazil, Sci Total Environ, p 139765

The manufacturer's authorised representative in the EU is Springer Nature Customer Service Centre GmbH, Europaplatz 3, 69115 Heidelberg, Germany. If you have any concerns regarding our products, please contact ProductSafety@springernature.com

Printed and bound by CPI Group (UK) Ltd, Croydon, CR0 4YY
30/09/2026
02225261-0014